Clinical Neurology: Essential Concepts

Clinical Neurology: Essential Concepts

Simon J. Ellis MA MB BChir MRCP MD

Consultant Neurologist and Senior Clinical Lecturer, North Staffordshire Royal Infirmary and Keele University

former Clinical Lecturer in Neurology at the University of Oxford

former Chief Resident in Neurology at Mount Sinai Medical Center, New York

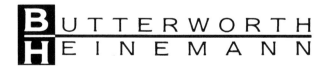
BUTTERWORTH
HEINEMANN

Butterworth-Heinemann
Linacre House, Jordan Hill, Oxford OX2 8DP
A division of Reed Educational and Professional Publishing Ltd

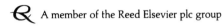 A member of the Reed Elsevier plc group

OXFORD   BOSTON   JOHANNESBURG
MELBOURNE   NEW DELHI   SINGAPORE

First published 1998

© Reed Educational and Professional Publishing Ltd 1998

British Library Cataloguing in Publication Data
A catalogue record for this book is available from the British Library

Library of Congress Cataloguing in Publication Data
A catalogue record for this book is available from the Library of Congress

ISBN 0 7506 3343 3

Data manipulation and artwork drawings by David Gregson Associates, Beccles, Suffolk
Printed and bound in Great Britain by The Alden Press, Oxford

Contents

Dedication

I would like to dedicate this book to the thousands of patients who have faced discomfort, disability and death with greater fortitude and courage than is ever seen on any battlefield; who have taught me the little neurology I know. In addition I would like to thank Melvin Yahr and the phenomenologists at Mount Sinai who have inspired me to love neurology with a passion.

Aus Liebe

Prologue

Objectives

Each chapter in this book has a series of objectives identified at the beginning.

    The overall objective of the book is to:

- Provide a good grounding in clinical neurology
- Make linkages with basic neuroscience
- Give clinical histories to make the pathology 'real'
- To explain the terminology

There have been two main spurs to writing this book; first, the difficulties medical students have with one of the most fascinating aspects of medicine and, second, the appalling standard of neurology practised in general medical firms. Four years of teaching neurology at Oxford demonstrated to me how ineffective didactic teaching is at imparting simple concepts. When I was at medical school I was taught that medical students can remember one fact in one hour and this certainly fits with my own experience when teaching. The primary purpose of this book is to teach facts. Reading alone is not sufficient. We have all read an article and on reaching the end wondered what it was all about. The durability of memory is dependent on the depth of processing.

I have structured the book into a 3-week course in neurology consisting of 20 chapters. At the end of each chapter there are multiple choice questions. The MCQs will encourage deeper processing and check retention. Of course there is no reason why this book could not be read over a longer period to allow for weekends off and a few days for quiet reflection on the meaning of life. I have tried to limit the material in the book to that which is clinically useful. Occasionally I have failed in this, tempted by some of the more exciting esoterica. But, primarily this book is written for the average medical student. My apologies to high flyers, you will not find much about Vogt–Koyanagi–Harada syndrome here. I have had to simplify some things in order to get across central concepts. I have also indulged in some neuromythology. I hope I have identified in the text wherever I have done this. If physicists can believe that a photon is both a wave and a particle at the same time then I have little problem believing in conduction aphasia.

Like all professionals neurologists have developed their own complex, opaque and exclusive terminology. Half the struggle in understanding a new field of knowledge is understanding the language. As well as an index I have included a glossary to facilitate this process.

I have used three neurological text books to check facts; *Neurology in Clinical Practice* (edited by WG Bradley, RB Daroff, GM Fenichel and CD Marsden, Butterworth-Heinemann, 1989), *Brain's Disease of the Nervous System* (edited by J Walton, Oxford University Press, 1993) and *Office Practice of*

Neurology (edited by MA Samuels and S Feske, Churchill Livingstone, 1996).

How to use this book

This book can either be dipped into via the index or can be used as a structured course. If it is being used as the latter I suggest that each day you read a chapter, making notes on it. On finishing the chapter do the MCQs at the end of that chapter. If you score greater than 60% then you have finished for the day. If you have not, reread the chapter and do the MCQs again until you do score more than 60%. At the end of the book do the final MCQs and you should score more than 50%. By doing the MCQs you will retain more information and they will act as an assessment of how much you have understood.

This book will not make you a good neurologist. For that you need empathy with your patients, an ability to communicate, a touch of obsessive compulsive disorder and years of experience. However, without a good knowledge base all the empathy on the planet will not help your patients. This book can give you a good knowledge base.

Acknowledgements

I would like to thank Alex Dombrowe and Helen Deane for proof reading this book, my editors Melanie Tait, Tim Brown and Geoffrey Smaldon at Butterworth-Heinemann for their support and encouragement and Andrea Nemeth for advice on genetics.

1. Introduction to neurology

Objectives

This chapter introduces neurology. A methodology for approaching a patient is given. The following areas are discussed:

- The philosophical basis of making a diagnosis
- Four questions that help in localization
- The concept of upper versus lower motor neurone
- Localization within the peripheral nervous system
- Localization in the central nervous system

By the end of this chapter you will have a passing familiarity with the whole of the neuroaxis.

Neurology has the reputation of being difficult. This is a myth perpetuated by neurologists for perfectly understandable reasons and by general physicians, because they feel insecure in their neurological knowledge. The understanding of any field of human knowledge can be likened to a tree with the facts being the leaves and the trunk and branches being the central concepts. A pile of leaves is a mess; a tree is an organized structure. Once you have an appreciation of the underlying structure the whole makes sense. The basics of neurology are simple. If you start from simple concepts and hang your knowledge on these then your task in becoming comfortable and competent in neurology should be easy.

The major challenge and joy in neurology is in making a diagnosis. The first principle we use in this endeavour is Occam's razor, 'What can be done with fewer (assumptions) is done in vain with more' (Ockham or Occam, William 1285–1350). This is also known as the law of parsimony, 'the principle that no more causes should be assumed than will account for the effect'. In the context of clinical medicine we presume that there is a single cause (diagnosis) and deduce the differential diagnosis from the causes that could give rise to that particular clinical picture. This works well for most patients where a single pathological process is active, but gives rise to great confusion when two or more are present, for example in the elderly.

In some neurological patients the diagnosis is obvious, however in many, more thought is required. The traditional approach to the neurological patient is to first make an anatomical diagnosis and then make a pathophysiological one. This continues to be a useful approach as it narrows the differential diagnosis considerably. To do this it is useful to ask oneself four questions:

1. **Is it neurological?**

2. **Is it central or peripheral?**

3. **Is it above or below the foramen magnum?**

4. **Is it above or below the tentorium?**

These questions allow one to focus the analysis of the patient's symptoms and signs and to make an anatomical diagnosis.

1. Is it neurological?

This is a useful question to raise at the start of the analysis. Many patients will present with physical symptoms which are psychological in origin and many will have psychological sounding symptoms which are physical in origin. Many patients will have both. Some readers will have questioned the distinction between psychological and physical. However, this difference is one of those myths that makes life for the neurologist possible. As well as differentiating the psychological from the neurological, cardiological and endocrinological causes of cerebral dysfunction have to be considered (e.g. cardiac arrhythmia as a cause of loss of consciousness).

2. Is it central or peripheral?

This is more or less the same as asking the difference between upper and lower motor neurone lesions.

There are four main characteristics of lower motor neurone lesions:

1. Profound wasting of muscle

2. Hyporeflexia (neuromythology)

3. Fasciculations

4. Reduced or normal tone.

The *profound wasting of muscle* seen in lower motor neurone lesions is a result of the loss of the trophic factor to muscle supplied by nerves.

Although *hyporeflexia* has traditionally been thought of as a lower motor neurone sign, in truth it is more often due to disturbance of the sensory arm of the reflex arc. Dispersion of the barrage of impulses arriving from the stretch receptors is a very effective way of producing hyporeflexia or areflexia (e.g. Guillian–Barré syndrome).

A *fasciculation* is the spontaneous firing of a motor unit. A motor unit is an α-motor neurone and all the muscle fascicules attached to it. The number of fascicules per α-motor neurone is inversely related to the degree of fine control required. Gastrocnemius may have 100 fascicules per neurone while hand muscles may have a one-to-one relationship. Fasciculations are seen more easily in the larger power muscles than the smaller fine control muscles. In slowly progressive denervating conditions motor units get larger as denervated fascicules join the surviving motor units. When one of these units becomes sick and the α-motor neurone starts firing spontaneously the resulting fasciculation will be larger and more easily seen (e.g. motor neurone disease). Normal people can have occasional fasciculations, particularly after drinking coffee. Do not make the mistake I made of thinking I had motor neurone disease on the basis of a few twitches!

If the lesion is in that desert of the intellect, the peripheral nervous system, some structure is necessary to localize the pathology and the easiest is anatomical, starting proximally and working distally:

1. Is it root (radiculopathy)? These are often painful with sensory disturbances that follow dermatomes.
2. Is it plexus? The pattern of sensory and motor deficits is too complex to be analysed in terms of roots or nerves.
3. Is it nerve(s)? Sensory abnormalities from single nerves are fairly simple to identify. When there is a generalized assault on all peripheral nerves, usually the longest nerves fail first, hence the glove and stocking sensory disturbance (though a similar sensory disturbance can be seen with cervical cord pathology, e.g. MS).
4. Is it neuromuscular junction? There should be no sensory involvement. The hallmark of neuromuscular junction dysfunction is fatiguability.
5. Is it muscle? Again there should be no sensory involvement apart from pain. Most weakness is worse proximally than distally in the limbs. There are three sorts of muscle pathology:

Dystrophies – genetically determined progressive atrophy of muscle, usually in children.

Myositises – inflammation in muscles with tenderness, worse proximally.
Myopathies – often biochemical/hormonal in origin, muscles not tender, worse proximally.

Let us now return to the question of lower versus upper motor neurone pathology. There are four main characteristics of an upper motor neurone lesion.

1. Hyper-reflexia
2. Increased tone
3. Little wasting
4. Primitive reflexes.

The commonest primitive reflex is Babinski's response. Others are the grasp, snout and root reflexes and the glabellar tap. These reflexes are suppressed by the phylogenetically more recent pyramidal system, but become apparent when that system is dysfunctional.

The central versus peripheral distinction is not exactly the same as the upper versus lower motor neurone differentiation. If there is evidence of an upper motor neurone lesion then there is central pathology, but the converse is not always correct. The cell body and proximal part of the axon of the α-motor neurone (the most common type of motor nerve) lie within the central nervous system. The majority lie in the cord, but neurones from the facial nerve are located in the brain stem. If a patient has a brain-stem stroke the facial weakness may well be of a lower motor neurone type. If the patient has a cord lesion, at the level of the cord pathology lower motor neurone signs can be found (e.g. syringomyelia). So central nervous system pathology can result in lower motor neurone signs.

neurone signs below the lesion. Though this may take some time to develop (spinal shock).

2. Sensation is abnormal below the level of the lesion. This has to be specifically looked for by testing for alterations in pin prick sensation up each side of the trunk.

3. There is autonomic dysfunction below the lesion. One has to ask specifically about bowel, bladder and sexual dysfunction including questions on continence and urgency.

When half the cord is damaged the pattern of motor and sensory dysfunction resulting is called the Brown–Séquard syndrome. In medical text books this consists of ipsilateral weakness, contralateral reduction in temperature and pain perception (spinothalamic) and ipsilateral loss of vibration and joint position sense (posterior column). In the real world one is presented with a patient with a weak leg but with better pin prick sensation in that leg as compared to the other. Usually this causes confusion until you think of Brown–Séquard syndrome. The resulting feeling of enlightenment is metaphysical in intensity.

● tentorium: extension of the dura matter that seperates the cerebellum from the inferior portion of the occipital lobes

4. ... in the posteri... ontains the cer... mesencephal... unction of these...

Nausea, vomiting, vertigo and nystagmus
Unsteadiness and loss of co-ordination in the limbs
Neighbourhood signs
Crossed motor and sensory syndromes
Pre-terminal drowsiness, coma, cardiovascular instability and respiratory failure.

Vertigo is often called dizziness by patients, but this term can be used to describe almost any neurological symptom. The term vertigo in

● foramen magnum: large opening in the occipital bone of the cranium.

...w the ...? ...e spinal cord is ...ain features of ...y bilateral, 'both ...th upper motor

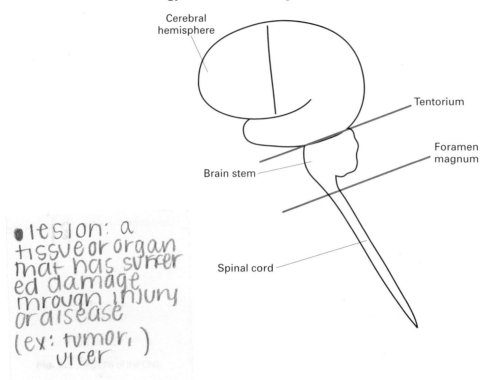

Handwritten note:
● lesion: a tissue or organ that has suffered damage through injury or disease (ex: tumor, ulcer)

a neurological sense refers to the hallucination of either the world or the individual moving in space, usually in a rotational axial plane.

Neighbourhood signs are the result of the brain stem being a crowded neighbourhood and consist of cranial nerve signs. The commonest being diplopia, dysarthria, dysphagia or sensory or motor disturbance of the face.

Crossed syndromes occur when there is a motor disturbance on one side of the face and in the contralateral arm and leg, or a sensory disturbance on one side of the face and in the opposite side of the body. This is due to the fact that the fibres supplying the face decussate at a higher level than the pyramids or the lemnisci, resulting in the possibility of these disassociations. These syndromes are rare, but very helpful in terms of localization.

It is not enough to have excluded the rest of the nervous system and therefore to conclude that the lesion is above the tentorium. This part of the nervous system includes that pinnacle of evolutionary effort, the neocortex.

Positive features pointing to dysfunction above the tentorium are given below.

Disorders of language (aphasias)
Loss of memory (usually temporal lobes)
Complex sensory dysfunction (steriognosis, graphaesthesiae)
Disorders of spatial function, visuospatial neglect
Homonymous hemianopsia
Loss of social inhibition and planning capacities (e.g. Phineas Gage).

A hemiplegia involving the face, arm and leg on the same side is most likely due to lesions in the internal capsule or motor cortex, but rarely can be due to pathology as low as the top of the pons. Thus this common constellation does not provide conclusive evidence of dysfunction above the tentorium.

In this chapter we have considered the whole of the nervous system and how to localize lesions within it. This is the basis of clinical neurology. Know this and you are halfway to being a competent neurologist.

MCQs for Chapter 1

The MCQs are either true T or false F. The answers are given in Appendix 3. Negatively mark your answers; a point for a correct answer, deduct a point for an incorrect response. If you score 24 or more you pass.

1. **The four questions I suggest are used to make an anatomical diagnosis are:**
   A Is it psychological?
   B Is it central or peripheral?
   C Is it above or below the foramen magnum?
   D Is it above or below the pons?

2.
   A Radiculopathies are often painful.
   B Glove and stocking sensory loss is pathognomonic for peripheral neuropathy.
   C Fatiguability is a hallmark of neuromuscular disorders.
   D Myositises usually occur in children.

3.
   A The principle of Occum's razor works well in the elderly.
   B Traditionally a pathophysiological diagnosis precedes an anatomical one.
   C Weakness of the face, arm and leg localizes the lesion to the internal capsule.
   D Coma is a feature of posterior fossa dysfunction.

4. **Features of lower motor neurone lesions found on examination are:**
   A Profound muscle wasting.
   B Hyper-reflexia.
   C Fibrillations.
   D Reduced or normal muscle tone.

5. **In spinal cord disease:**
   A Usually both legs are weak.
   B Sensation is abnormal above the lesion.

   C Urgency of micturition is not a feature.
   D Impotence can be a feature.

6. **Features of posterior fossa dysfunction are:**
   A Neighbourhood signs.
   B Vomiting.
   C Crossed sensory dysfunction.
   D Aphasia.

7. **The cardinal features of upper motor neurone pathology are:**
   A Hyporeflexia.
   B Increased tone.
   C Unilateral sensory loss.
   D Primitive reflexes.

8.
   A Lower motor neurone signs can occur with CNS pathology.
   B Syringomyelia is often associated with lower motor neurone signs.
   C The Babinski response is a normal variant.
   D Upper motor neurone signs can be due to peripheral lesions.

9. **In the Brown–Séquard syndrome:**
   A Weakness is ipsilateral to the lesion.
   B Pin prick loss is contralateral to the lesion.
   C Vibration and joint position sense loss is contralateral to the lesion.
   D Is due to hemisection of the corpus callosum.

10. **Features of dysfunction above the tentorium are:**
    A Visuospatial neglect.
    B Homonimous hemianopia.
    C Nystagmus.
    D Memory loss.

Common presentations

2. Headache

Objectives

In this chapter you will become acquainted with the clinical features and learn about the management of:

- Raised intracranial pressure
- Headache of temporal (giant cell) arteritis
- Migraine
- Cluster headache
- Benign sex headache
- Cervical spondylosis
- Sinusitis
- Trigeminal neuralgia
- Atypical facial pain
- Non-specific (tension-type) headache
- Chronic daily headache

Basic science – 5-HT (serotonin)

Headache is an almost ubiquitous human experience. It ranges from the occasional 'rough head' after excessive alcohol to a severely debilitating daily event. Headache is the most common reason for seeking neurological advice. The usual concern behind the referral is the fear of raised intracranial pressure due to an underlying brain tumour. Sudden severe headaches cause considerable anxiety in patients and their attending doctors and though the majority will be benign, any headache of a severe nature and of sudden onset should be presumed to be subarachnoid haemorrhage until proven otherwise. The main characteristics of some of the headache syndromes are given in Table 2.1. As with the majority of medicine, the key to the diagnosis is good history taking.

Headache of raised intracranial pressure (ICP)

Classically this is a dull frontal headache, worse in the mornings, associated with nausea and exacerbated by Valsalva manoeuvres such as coughing or straining. There may be visual obscurations and false localizing signs such as a sixth nerve palsy. Papilloedema is a late and unreliable sign. The headache initially responds to minor analgesics. The classical picture of a raised intracranial pressure headache is rare and all practising neurologists have diagnosed raised ICP as migraine or tension headache only to be proven incorrect by the scan. Usually it is associated features, such as focal neurological deficits, blunting of intellec-

Raised intracranial pressure
Frontal
Nausea and vomiting
Worse in the mornings
Visual obscurations
Gradually getting worse over weeks
Migraine
Often unilateral
Nausea and vomiting
Visual phenomena (positive and negative)
Lasts hours at a time
Family history
Non-specific (tension-type) headache
A band round the head or bitemporal
Always present for weeks at a time
Exacerbated by stress
Temporal arteritis
Scalp tenderness (brushing hair painful)
Jaw claudication
Present for weeks
Uniocular visual change
Magical response to steroids
Subarachnoid haemorrhage
Sudden onset (seconds)
Severe (worst headache of their life)
Angor animi (fear of imminent doom)
Nausea and vomiting
Loss of consciousness
Subsequent neck stiffness and photophobia

Table 2.1 Characteristics of the more important headache syndromes

tual faculties and rarely papilloedema, that alert the clinician to the diagnosis. While clinical machismo is fine for grand rounds patients rarely benefit from it and most neurologists have a low threshold for ordering a CT scan of the head. However, a headache that has been present for over a year or is unilateral and episodic is unlikely to be due to raised ICP.

Headache of temporal (giant cell) arteritis

This condition is covered in more detail in Chapter 15. However, this diagnosis should be considered in anyone over 50 presenting with headache. The main clue as to the diagnosis is that the scalp is tender, so the patient has difficulty brushing their hair or laying their head on a pillow at night. An ESR is a rapid and relatively good screening test.

Migraine

Over 10% of the population suffer with migraine. There is nearly always a family history and the disorder usually starts in adolescence or in the twenties. The two most frequent sorts are classical and common. The modern classification is migraine with aura (classical) and migraine without aura (common). Classical migraine often starts with an aura. The aura is often visual, but can involve any neurological function. Initially there may be positive phenomena, such as flashing lights or coloured zig-zag lines (fortification spectra) which are followed by negative phenomena such as scotoma (holes in the visual fields). About half an hour after the start of the aura the headache arrives. This is usually unilateral, severe and associated with nausea, vomiting, phonophobia and photophobia. Most patients take analgesia and go to bed in a darkened room. Sleep is often beneficial. The attack will last from hours to a whole day. Often the patient feels 'hung over' the next day. Common migraine is the same but without the aura.

Other types of migraine are vertebrobasilar migraine where the symptomatology is attributable to the posterior fossa, retinal migraine where the visual loss is explicable in retinal terms (one eye only), and hemiplegic migraine, where a hemiplegia is associated with the migraine. Complicated migraine is said to occur when the neurological deficits are semipermanent. CT scanning will demonstrate ischaemic damage in complicated migraine.

Stress, or relief of stress, can precipitate migraine as can certain foods, particularly cheese, chocolate and red wine. Treatment can be divided into acute and prophylactic. The simplest acute treatment is with minor analgesics often in combination with an antiemetic. This is most effective if given early in the attack. Two aspirin and two paracetamols at the first inkling of an attack is a safe and

Case history

Mrs Fenton is a 35-year-old housewife with three children and a part-time cleaning job. During childhood she would have 'bilious attacks' which would consist of episodes of nausea and feeling generally unwell. This would result in her taking time off school. At 16 she had her first attack of her usual headaches. These attacks started with scintillations in one half of the visual field which would be followed by the development of a scotoma. This would resolve over a quarter of an hour, but 20 minutes later she would develop a severe unilateral headache centred behind an eye associated with nausea and vomiting. The pain could be over either side of the head, but was usually on the right. She would have photophobia and phonophobia and lie down in a darkened room. The worst of the attack would last from 3 to 4 hours, but she would have a headache for the rest of the day and the next day she would be 'out of sorts'. The attacks would occur about twice a month, often in the week before her period. She would take paracetamol/opiate analgesics, which were of benefit if she took them at the start of the attack, but were ineffective once the attack was established. Her attacks could be precipitated by red wine, but not chocolate or cheese. There had been a marked increase in the frequency of her attacks around the time of her divorce. Her mother had suffered from similar episodes and Emma, her 12-year-old, was developing 'bilious attacks'.

pizotifen causes weight gain. Pizotifen and propanolol often fail because too low a dosage is given for too short a time. Pizotifen should be started at 1.5 mg at night and continued for at least 3 weeks, then increased to 3 mg at night. Propanolol should be built up to between 80 and 160 mg a day. Amitriptyline is used at 10–25 mg at night which is well below its antidepressant dosage. It has the advantage of often being effective in non-specific (tension) headache.

Rarely, migraine can be symptomatic of an underlying vascular anomaly such as an arteriovenous malformation or an aneurysm. It is difficult to identify these patients out of the hosts of idiopathic migrainers, but a lack of a family history, late onset, pain localized only to one side of the head and never on the other side, and migraine resistant to treatment are all pointers.

Status migrainosus is the situation when one migraine runs into the next so the patient is in a constant headache state for weeks at a time. This often responds to 24 hours of adequate opiate analgesia to break the status followed by one of the prophylactic agents. In general, long-term opiates should be avoided not only because of their addictive potential, but because they tend to produce rebound headaches.

cheap ploy. If that is insufficient sumatriptan (a 5-HT agonist) either orally or subcutaneously is often effective. Ergotamines have fallen from favour because of the dangers of ergotism in overdosage, but should not be forgotten for those in whom sumatriptan is ineffective or not tolerated. Patients who have one or two disabling attacks per month should be considered for prophylaxis. There are three effective and commonly used drugs for prophylaxis; they are propanolol, pizotifen and amitriptyline. Propanolol cannot be given if there is a history of cardiac failure or asthma,

Cluster headache

This term is often used incorrectly to describe a few migraines occurring together over a few days. Cluster headache is very specific and consists of a severe pain over one eye lasting between 20 minutes and an hour, which tends to reoccur at the same time each day. The pain is frequently associated with reddening of the eye, tearing and filling of the nostril on that side. The pain is so severe that otherwise rational people consider suicide. The pains reoccur daily for up to 6 weeks at a time and then disappear for months or years only to reoccur. This is why it is called cluster.

Basic science – 5-HT (serotonin)

Serotonin (5-Hydroxytryptamine) is one of the major neurotransmitters. Others include dopamine, acetylcholine, GABA, glycine, glutamate and aspartate. 5-HT is structurally similar to LSD. It is synthesized from tryptophan and is broken down by monoamine oxidase. There are large amounts in the pineal and clusters of cells containing 5-HT are found in the midline or raphe regions of the pons and upper brain stem. 5-HT produces its effects mainly by inhibition. It is involved in migraine, depression, anxiety, obsessive compulsive disorder, obesity and nausea and vomiting. The complexity of 5-HT pharmacology relates to the plethora of receptor types. The important receptors from a clinical point of view are 5-HT_{1A}, 5-HT_{1C}, 5-HT_{1D}, 5-HT_2, and 5-HT_3. The SSRI group of antidepressants (fluoxetine [Prozac], sertraline [Lustral]) block uptake of 5-HT and are used in the treatment of depression, obsessive compulsive disorder and bulimia nervosa. Buspirone is a partial agonist on 5-HT_{1A} receptors and is used to treat anxiety. Lithium likewise acts on 5-HT_{1A} as an agonist and is used in manic depression and occasionally in refractory headache. Pizotifen and methysergide, both used in migraine prophylaxis, are $5\text{-HT}_{1\&2}$ antagonists. The antidepressant mianserin is a 5-HT_{1C} receptor antagonist. Effective acute migraine treatment is often provided by sumatriptan (Imigran) which is a 5-HT_{1D} agonist. The hallucinogen LSD is a partial agonist of 5-HT_2 receptors. Ondansetron, which is used as an antiemetic during chemotherapy, is a 5-HT_3 receptor antagonist. Fenfluramine, an appetite suppressant, and MDMA (the recreational drug ecstasy), have their effects on 5-HT release. Fenfluramine increases release and blocks re-uptake, and MDMA increases release. 5-HT, with its associations with agony and ecstasy, may be truly described as a mind-bending neurotransmitter.

Treatment consists of sumatriptan injections or inhaled oxygen for the acute attacks, pizotifen, steroids and/or lithium as prophylaxis during the cluster.

Benign sex headache

This is not the same as the headache that either sex can miraculously develop in order to avoid a sexual encounter. This headache is most unwelcome. It occurs just at the point of orgasm and is sudden and severe, and persists in a milder form for a number of hours. It can occur in either gender and seems to be a form of exertional headache. On the first occasion it cannot be differentiated clinically from a subarachnoid haemorrhage. If the patient has had many similar attacks the diagnosis can be made with confidence. Treatment is with reassurance that there is no serious underlying pathology and that these headaches spontaneously disappear over the next few weeks. Indomethacin has been used as prophylaxis.

Cervical spondylosis

Degenerative disease of the cervical spine is ubiquitous as patients grow older. Not infrequently the cervical roots that supply the back of the head become involved, giving rise to pain in the occipital region which may be exacerbated by neck movements. Treatment is with non-steroidal anti-inflammatories and physiotherapy.

Sinusitis

Sinusitis often causes a chronic frontal headache. It can be detected clinically by eliciting tenderness on percussing over the sinuses. The diagnosis can be confirmed with plane skull films or more sensitively by CT of the sinuses. Treatment is initially with analgesics, antibiotics and decongestants.

Trigeminal neuralgia

Trigeminal neuralgia is a lancinating (short duration) pain in the distribution of one of the divisions of the trigeminal nerve (usually the second or third). It is often triggered by touch, chewing or even a breath of wind. The pain is severe and occurs hundreds of times a day. As the disorder continues the pain can become more persistent. In younger people it can be secondary to multiple sclerosis. In the older population, in whom it is more common, it is usually idiopathic. Carbamazepine is usually effective in controlling it, though dosages associated with drowsiness are often needed. Phenytoin, valproate and lamotrigine are less effective alternatives. If the condition fails to respond to medical treatment and does not spontaneously remit, various surgical interventions are available, either to move blood vessels from compressing the trigeminal nerve or to damage the trigeminal ganglion.

Atypical facial pain

Atypical facial pain consists of pain in the face which is not attributable to any other pathological process such as dental trouble or temporomandibular joint problems. It is usually chronic and sometimes responds to low dose amitriptyline.

Non-specific headache (tension-type headache)

Non-specific headache is more commonly known as tension headache or tension-type headache. Classically it consists of a band of pain around the head or bitemporal boring pains. It is supposed to be exacerbated by stress. It is probably one end of a spectrum of vascular headaches with classical migraine at the other end. Paracetamol and NSAIDs are frequently used by patients, but are not very effective and can lead to chronic daily headache. Non-specific headache often responds to reassurance and low dose amitriptyline.

Chronic daily headache

Patients who suffer headache every day, or most days of a month, have chronic daily headache. Many forms of headache can become transformed into chronic daily headache. The major cause for the transformation being drug misuse. Minor analgesics, opiates, ergotamine and even sumatriptan can cause this problem. The medication relieves the acute headache, but the patient develops a rebound headache as the medication wears off, so takes more. This vicious cycle then repeats itself. The mainstay of treatment is explanation to the patient and withdrawal of excessive drug usage.

MCQs for Chapter 2

The MCQs are either true T or false F. The answers are given in Appendix 3. Negatively mark your answers; a point for a correct answer, deduct a point for an incorrect response. If you score 24 or more you pass.

1. **Features of raised intracranial pressure include:**
   A Nausea and vomiting.
   B Fortification spectra.
   C Headaches worse in the mornings.
   D Unilateral headaches.

2. **Features of temporal arteritis include:**
   A Scalp tenderness.
   B Slow response to steroids.
   C Jaw claudication.
   D Sudden onset headache.

3. **Prophylactic therapies for migraine include:**
   A Sumatriptan.
   B Ergotamines.
   C Pizotifen.
   D Amitriptyline.

4. **Cluster headache**
   A Is associated with reddening of the eye.
   B Is associated with filling of the nostril.
   C Is a continuous pain for weeks at a time.
   D Is associated with thoughts of suicide.

5. **Trigeminal neuralgia**
   A Is always idiopathic.
   B Paracetamol is a good first line therapy.
   C Initially the pain is lancinating.
   D Is often triggered by cheese.

6. **Migraine**
   A Commonly is associated with a family history.
   B Onset is usually after the age of 40.
   C Stress may precipitate it.
   D Is rarely associated with nausea and vomiting.

7. **Precipitants of migraine include:**
   A Red wine.
   B Cheese.
   C Sleep.
   D Relief of stress.

8. **Acute treatments of migraine include:**
   A Paracetamol.
   B Methysergide.
   C Aspirin.
   D Inhaled oxygen.

9. **Serotonin.**
   A 5-HT is broken down by COMT.
   B 5-HT is found in the upper brain stem.
   C Fluoxetine blocks the re-uptake of 5-HT.
   D MDMA blocks 5-HT release.

10. **Chronic daily headache**
    A Is usually a transformed headache.
    B Is often iatrogenic.
    C Opiate usage can precipitate it.
    D It responds to ergotamines.

3. Transient loss of consciousness

Objectives

In this chapter the clinical approach to a patient with transient loss of consciousness will be examined. The presentations of the following are discussed:

- Funny turns
- Cardiac arrhythmia
- Vasovagal syncope
- Postural hypotension
- Epilepsy

Basic science – the reticular activating system

Funny turns

Funny turns are a frequent problem in neurological practice. The usual question is whether the attacks are epileptic in origin or not. Epilepsy is discussed in detail in Chapter 16. It is very helpful to have an eye witness account of the attacks, but usually the patients themselves can give a lot of valuable information. The patient should be asked to give a second by second account of their recollection of the attack and its aftermath. Witnesses should then give their account. The most important indicators to the diagnosis are given in Table 3.1. The most important question is whether the patient lost consciousness or not. If they did then the differential diagnosis is given in Table 3.2. As usual the most powerful investigative tool is a detailed history, but the measuring of lying and standing blood pressure is a useful and neglected adjunct. In general, investigations have a low yield. However, ECG, EEG, CT of the head, and 24-hour ECG need to be considered. Thought has to be given before ordering an investigation. If clinically the patient does not have epilepsy

then it is a mistake to do an EEG as 1% of the normal population have an epileptogenic-appearing EEG and such a finding might encourage an incorrect diagnosis. It is better to call an attack an episode of loss of consciousness of unknown aetiology and to await events than to mislabel a patient.

Approach to the patient with loss of consciousness

As in all neurology the most important aspect is the history. First take a good history, second, take a good history and, third, take a good history. At medical school we are taught to use open questions to allow the patient to express themselves. This is a useful opening gambit, but most neurologists will use a series of highly directed questions to obtain the information they need to make a diagnosis (Table 3.3): What were the circumstances under which this occurred? Had anything out of the ordinary happened in the previous 24–48 hours? Had you been to a party/stayed up late/used recreational drugs? What was the first thing you noticed out of the ordinary? What happened next? And then what hap-

Loss of consciousness
Cardiac arrhythmia
Vasovagal syncope
Postural hypotension
Epilepsy
Always on standing
Vasovagal syncope
Postural hypotension
Warning
Aura
    2° generalized epilepsy
Pre-syncope
    Cardiac arrhythmia
    Vasovagal syncope
    Postural hypotension
Palpitation
Tachyarrhythmia
Anxiety/panic attack
Prolonged recovery (postictal) phase
Epilepsy
Tongue biting and urinary incontinence
Generalized epilepsy

Table 3.1 How to sort out funny turns

Idiopathic
Postural hypotension
Vasovagal syncope
Hypovolaemia
    Drugs (diuretics)
    Haemorrhage (e.g. GIT)
    Dehydration (e.g. D&V)
Autonomic failure
    Drugs (β-blockers)
    Autonomic neuropathy (DM)
    Central (Shy–Drager)
Cardiac
    Arrhythmias
    Tachyarrythmias
    Bradyarrhythmias
Pump failure
Seizures
Epilepsy
    Primary generalized
        Tonic-clonic
        Absence
    Secondary generalized
    Partial complex
Non-epileptic seizure disorder
Transient ischaemic attack (TIA) – Vertebrobasilar
    distribution
Raised intracranial pressure
    Subarachnoid haemorrhage
    Intracerebral haemorrhage
Head trauma
Biochemical, e.g. hypoglycaemia

Table 3.2 Differential diagnosis of transient loss of consciousness

pened? When you woke up how did you feel? Had you bitten your tongue (painful) or wet yourself? Were you confused? Did you have a headache or were you tired? Did your muscles ache? How long did it take you to get back to normal?

An eye witness account is very useful, particularly when someone loses consciousness. Patients will often not bring along an eye witness; however, they are usually available on the telephone and a simple call will usually obtain the information required. If that fails then the witness can be invited to come along to the next appointment.

Cardiac arrhythmia

Cardiac arrhythmias can occur at any age, but are commoner in patients at risk of ischaemic heart disease. They divide into tachyarrhythmias and bradyarrhythmias. Tachyarrhythmias may be associated with palpitation and/or chest pain prior to loss of consciousness. Both usually have feelings of presyncope pres-

ent prior to the loss of consciousness. Presyncope is the subjective sensation of cerebral hypoperfusion. It consists of a feeling that one is about to 'faint', 'dizziness' which is usually not true vertigo, and graying out of vision. These are the same symptoms most patients will be familiar with on initially standing after having had a hot bath. Cardiac arrhythmias occur in any position. Clues as to the aetiology may be found on the standard 12-lead ECG, such as degrees of heart block or a δ wave (as in Wolf–Parkinson–White syndrome). In addition, a 24-hour ECG may show short runs of abnormal rhythm. Not infrequently more than one 24-hour ECG is needed or specialist cardiological electrophysiological investigations.

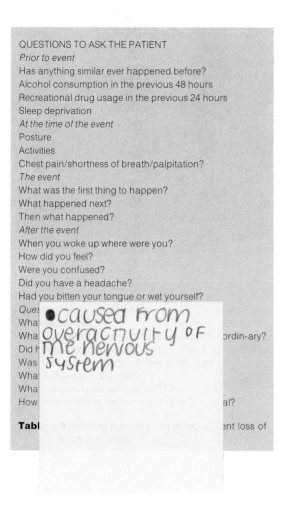

QUESTIONS TO ASK THE PATIENT
Prior to event
Has anything similar ever happened before?
Alcohol consumption in the previous 48 hours
Recreational drug usage in the previous 24 hours
Sleep deprivation
At the time of the event
Posture
Activities
Chest pain/shortness of breath/palpitation?
The event
What was the first thing to happen?
What happened next?
Then what happened?
After the event
When you woke up where were you?
How did you feel?
Were you confused?
Did you have a headache?
Had you bitten your tongue or wet yourself?
Ques...
Wha... ●caused from
Wha... overactivity of ...ordin-ary?
Did h... the nervous
Was... system
Wha...
Wha...
How... ...al?

Tabl... ...ent loss of

Vasovagal syncope

The term vasovagal syncope is used rather loosely, but refers to a physiological response to stimuli. It consists of overactivity of the parasympathetic nervous system with brady-cardia and vasodilatation resulting in a fall in blood pressure and cerebral hypoperfusion. This response can be precipitated by pain and emotional states. Sometimes on standing, after initial activation of the sympathetic nervous system, there can be a rebound over-activity of the parasympathetic. It is particularly common in adolescents. Vasovagal syncope can be investigated using a tilt table test. A similar condition is carotid sinus syndrome where tactile stimuli to the neck stimulates the carotid sinus resulting in syncope.

Case history

Paul Shelton is a 21-year-old architecture student who had been having a fairly wild time at university. Most weekends he would go night clubbing and use 'E'. While his weekends were excellent fun his weeks were getting to be less productive. He was having difficulty socializing with his fellow students and was becoming more isolated. During the week he felt low and would not want to go out. One Monday three weeks previously he had been walking around a meadow near his flat when he noticed the sunlight flickering through the trees. For a moment he felt strange and the next second he found himself lying on the wet grass. He had a headache and was slightly confused. Two months previously he had been walking down a street with tall iron railings at the side. The sun was shining through the railings and as he walked the light flickered across his face. He felt strange and his legs gave from under him. He did not completely collapse, but his ex-girlfriend had to help him back home. As a baby he had had two febrile convulsions.

This history is highly suggestive of epilepsy, probably precipitated by a combination of his ecstasy use and the photic stimulation of the sunlight. In addition, his life was beginning to suffer from his excessive use of ecstasy and he was developing a depressive illness. He was advised to moderate his recreational drug usage and avoid flickering lights. He had a single further episode of a strange feeling a couple of weeks later in a nightclub when a strobe light was used, but managed to get his life sorted out without recourse to psychiatrists or antiepileptic drugs.

Postural hypotension

On changing from a lying to a standing posture the vasculature has to undertake a number of changes in order to maintain cerebral perfusion. These changes consist of vasoconstriction and a slight speeding up of the heart. Postural hypotension occurs when these changes fail to occur and blood pools where gravity says it should, in the legs. Cardiac return falls, so does cardiac output, resulting in a fall in blood pressure and cerebral hypoperfusion. Postural hypotension is often due to drugs such as diuretics or β-blockers, but is also caused by damage to the autonomic nervous system as in diabetic autonomic neuropathy.

The first-aid solution both to postural hypotension and vasovagal syncope is to lie the patient flat and elevate the legs. This results in increased cerebral perfusion and rapid recovery.

In cardiac arrhythmias, vasovagal syncope and postural hypotension there is cerebral hypoperfusion so the patient experiences presyncope and looks deathly pale.

Epilepsy

Epilepsy is discussed in detail in Chapter 16. There are two main types of epilepsy, focal and primary generalized. In primary generalized the patient has no warning before loss of consciousness. In focal epilepsy there is an aura prior to loss of consciousness if the patient progresses to a secondary generalized seizure. Partial or focal seizures that do not progress to secondary generalized attacks are further subdivided into simple and complex. The term complex denotes some clouding of consciousness. Epilepsy can produce many different subjective experiences or behaviours. The commonest is the generalized seizure or grand mal fit. During this the patient may cry out, fall to the ground unconscious, go stiff all over and then shake in a violent fashion. There may be tongue biting or urinary incontinence. The patient then lies comatose for a period then gradually wakes up with a postictal period. During this time he/she is

> ### Basic science – the reticular activating system
>
> In order to lose consciousness either both cerebral hemispheres or the brain stem have to be involved in a pathological process. The reason the brain stem is so important in the maintenance of consciousness is the reticular activating system. Lesions in the rostral brain stem result in loss of consciousness and an EEG pattern similar to sleep ('The big sleep'). The reticular formation extends throughout the brain stem and is in continuity with the intralaminar nuclei of the thalamus. It is a loose collection of cells and fibres lying between the motor and sensory nuclei and tracts. It receives input from the spinoreticular tract and from the supraspinal system. The reticular formation controls the state of arousal and is important in autonomic reflex responses and in motivational and affective responses to stimuli.

confused and drowsy. The main hallmarks of epilepsy are that it is recurrent and stereotyped. It can occur in any posture.

Driving

The rules relating to epilepsy and driving are discussed in Chapter 16. However, any unexplained loss of consciousness results in disqualification from driving until the driver has been attack free for a year. If a diagnosis of vasovagal syncope can be made this stricture does not apply. The reason for this is simple, one is unlikely to be standing or in severe pain when driving. The driving regulations may be harsh, but they do contain a certain logic directed to the protection of patients and the general public.

MCQs for Chapter 3

The MCQs are either true T or false F. The answers are given in Appendix 3. Negatively mark your answers; a point for a correct answer, deduct a point for an incorrect response. If you score 24 or more you pass.

1. **Causes of loss of consciousness include:**
   A Postural hypotension.
   B Simple focal seizures.
   C Carotid distribution TIA.
   D Subarachnoid haemorrhage.

2. **Useful investigations in loss of consciousness include:**
   A 24-hour ECG.
   B CT scan of the head.
   C EMG.
   D PET scan.

3. **Episodes of loss of consciousness that occur on standing include:**
   A Myoclonic epilepsy.
   B Tachyarrhythmia.
   C Postural hypotension.
   D Vasovagal syncope.

4. **Types of loss of consciousness often preceded by a warning include:**
   A Vasovagal syncope.
   B Cardiac arrhythmia.
   C Secondary generalized epilepsy.
   D Absence (petit mal) epilepsy.

5. **Causes of hypovolaemia include:**
   A Cardiogenic shock.
   B Gastrointestinal haemorrhage.
   C Diarrhoea.
   D Syndrome of inappropriate ADH.

6. **Drugs causally linked to loss of consciousness include:**
   A Diuretics.
   B β–blockers.
   C Angiotensin converting enzyme inhibitors.
   D Insulin.

7. **Types of raised intracranial pressure associated with sudden loss of consciousness:**
   A Benign intracranial hypertension.
   B Subarachnoid haemorrhage.
   C Intracerebral haemorrhage.
   D Normal pressure hydrocephalus.

8. **Typical symptoms following a generalized tonic-clonic seizure include:**
   A Headache.
   B Thirst.
   C Euphoria.
   D Drowsiness.

9. **Useful questions to ask a patient who may have had a seizure include:**
   A How many cigarettes did you smoke the day before the event?
   B How much alcohol did you consume in the 48 hours before the event?
   C Do you smoke marihuana?
   D How much sleep did you get the night before the attack?

10. **Useful questions to ask a witness of a presumed seizure:**
    A What did he/she last have to eat?
    B Was he/she in pain?
    C Did he/she change colour?
    D How long did it take him/her to get back to normal?

4. Dizziness

Objectives

In this chapter the meaning of the symptom 'dizziness' is explored. Topics covered include:

- Vertigo
- Presyncopal dizziness
- Hypoglycaemic dizziness
- Psychogenic dizziness
- Drug-induced dizziness
- Disequilibrium

The Hallpike and modified Epley manoeuvres are explained.

Basic science – the vestibular system

Dizziness as a symptom

Dizziness means different things to different people. When a patient uses the term to describe their symptoms the exact meaning has to be identified. Usually one has to give the patient examples of the different sorts of dizziness, such as feelings of presyncope on getting out of a hot bath, vertigo after being on a roundabout and disequilibrium after excessive amounts of alcohol.

Vertigo

Vertigo is the hallucination that either the world or the subject is in motion when they are not. It usually consists of a feeling of rotation in the axial plane. The most common causes are acute labyrinthitis, benign positional vertigo, Menière's disease, benign recurrent vertigo, migraine and vertebrobasilar ischaemia.

Acute labyrinthitis

The symptoms of acute labyrinthitis consist of vertigo, nausea and vomiting, and an unsteadiness with a tendency to fall to one side. The patient may have marked nystagmus, particularly to one side. The condition will resolve over a few days. Treatment is symptomatic and supportive with prochlorperazine and metoclopramide for the nausea and dizziness. Sometimes patients become dehydrated through vomiting and require intravenous hydration. The condition is often attributed to a virus.

Benign positional vertigo

Benign positional vertigo (BPV) is a syndrome of sudden attacks of vertigo which are precipitated by a change of posture, such as turning in bed. Unfortunately, less benign forms of vertigo can be precipitated by alteration in posture. BPV is caused by calcium carbonate crystals within the posterior semicircular canal which land on the cupula,

Case history

June Penkhull is a 67-year-old retired fettler who was referred for an opinion on her 'dizziness'. Two years prior to being seen she had 3 days of dizziness where everything span round her head. She vomited several times and she had to hold onto the walls as she walked to the toilet. She made a complete recovery, but for the last 6 months she has had a similar spinning feeling in her head, particularly on getting up in the morning. Close questioning revealed that it was the act of sitting up in bed rather than standing that brought on her vertigo. In addition, when she lay down in bed at night she had an attack. Recently she had found that even if she turned in bed at night she would get attacks of vertigo that would wake her. Apart from obesity her examination was unremarkable. In particular, there was no deafness or nystagmus. How-ever, on performing the Hallpike manoeuvre she felt very unwell and 'dizzy' and nystagmus was induced both by lying her down and sitting her up.

The initial episode of vertigo which occurred 2 years previously could well have been an episode of labyrinthitis. The current problem is one of benign positional vertigo. She was reassured and a modified Epley manoeuvre was attempted with only partial success.

Vertigo
Acute labyrinthitis
Benign positional vertigo
Ménière's disease
Benign recurrent vertigo
Migraine
Vertebrobasilar ischaemia
Presyncopal dizziness
Postural hypotension
Vasovagal presyncope
Cardiac arrhythmia
Hypoglycaemic dizziness
Diabetes treated with insulin
Postgastric surgery
Alcoholism
Insulinoma
Psychogenic dizziness
Anxiety states
Phobias
Panic attacks
Drug-induced dizziness
Ethanol
Antiepileptic drugs
Tranquillizers
Disequilibrium
Cerebrovascular disease
Peripheral neuropathy
Ototoxicity
Cerebellar degeneration

Table 4.1 What dizziness means

resulting in a burst of nystagmus and vertigo. This can be demonstrated by the Hallpike maneuvre. It can be cured in up to 80% of cases by a modified Epley manoeuvre.

The Hallpike manoeuvre
The Hallpike manoeuvre is a serious misnomer. The paper usually quoted was by Dix and Hallpike but the original description of the phenomenon was by Bárány 31 years previously! The patient is sat on a couch and then rapidly laid down with the head hanging over the end of the couch at a 30° angle below the rest of the body. The head is also rotated 30–40° towards the observer. After a few seconds vertigo and nystagmus will occur in benign positional vertigo. The nystagmus is towards the lowest ear which is the affected one. The test can be repeated by rotating the head in the other direction to test the other ear. The symptoms reoccur on sitting the patient up.

The modified Epley manoeuvre
The Epley manoeuvre is used to treat BPV after the condition has been diagnosed using the Hallpike manoeuvre. In addition the Hallpike will have identified in which ear the calcium carbonate crystals lie. The patient is placed in a sitting position with the head rotated towards the side of the affected ear. The patient is then laid down with the head hanging at a 30° angle below the level of the couch with the head still rotated towards the affected ear. The head is then rapidly rotated in the opposite direction so the affected ear is now uppermost. This position is maintained for 30 seconds. The patient then lies on the side

with the unaffected ear downmost and the head remaining rotated towards that side. The nose will be towards the ground at this stage and the position should be maintained for 30 seconds. The patient is then rapidly sat up with the head rotated to the unaffected side. The cycle is repeated until no nystagmus is elicited. The patient is advised not to lie flat for the next 2 days to allow the debits to become fixed and not fall back into the posterior canal. This manoeuvre requires a little practice.

Ménière's disease

Ménière's disease consists of recurrent episodes of vertigo lasting a few hours to weeks in duration associated with gradual hearing loss and tinnitus. It is caused by idiopathic distension of the endolymphatic system. It is relatively common with a prevalence of 370/100 000. Treatment is with salt restriction, diuretics and vestibular sedatives such as prochlorperazine. Surgical intervention is reserved for refractory cases.

Basic science – the vestibular system

There are three main ways in which we maintain an upright position; through proprioceptive input from our legs, through visual input telling us where the horizontal is and through information on head position obtained from the vestibular system. It is one of the wonders of our bodies that minute movements of the head are detected and that information is used to tell us that our head has moved and not the San Andreas fault.

As well as the cochlea the inner ear consists of three semicircular canals set at right angles to each other. At the end of these canals is a dilatation called the ampulla in which lies the cupola and its hair cells. These cells respond to movement of the endolymph. These responses are sent down the vestibular nerve to the vestibula nuclei and eye movement nuclei in the brain stem. These signals inform the brain about movement of the head. In the utricle lies the otolith. This has a field of hair cells with calcium carbonate crystals on them. The messages from the otolith inform the brain about head tilt (Fig 4.1).

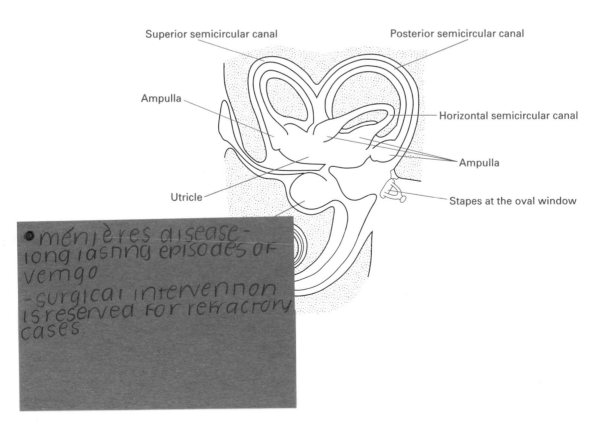

Superior semicircular canal — Posterior semicircular canal — Ampulla — Horizontal semicircular canal — Ampulla — Utricle — Stapes at the oval window

Benign recurrent vertigo

Episodes of vertigo lasting hours or days can occur which can be quite disabling. It is usually a diagnosis of exclusion. Clinically it can only be differentiated from Ménière's disease in retrospect in that hearing loss does not develop. Vestibular sedatives are usually given, though without much benefit.

Migraine

Ve   om of migraine. It is pr   in vertebrobasilar migraine. Other sy   re the classical ones of migraine including headache, nausea, vomiting, photophobia, phonophobia and mild encephalopathy. Vertebrobasilar migraine is a diagnostic trap as serious pathology in the posterior fossa needs excluding.

Vertebrobasilar ischaemia

Impairment of the blood supply as in a brainstem TIA/stroke or to the vestibular organs themselves can cause vertigo. Brain-stem TIA should not be diagnosed on the basis of vertigo alone. The brain stem is a crowded neighbourhood and in the vast majority of cases there will be other signs and symptoms such as visual disturbance, altered sensation or motor function, or a change in the level of consciousness.

Presyncopal dizziness

Postural hypotension results in hypoperfusion of the brain stem. Usually this gives a subjective feeling of faintness or light-headedness rather than true vertigo. Vasovagal syncope, which has been discussed in the previous chapter, gives rise to similar symptoms, but often with the addition of autonomic symptoms such as feeling hot and cold and sweaty. Cardiac arrhythmia can cause global cerebral hypoperfusion. If the arrhythmia is short-lived and does not compromise cardiac output too much then it may produce feelings of presyncope. If it is prolonged and/or impairs cardiac function sufficiently, arrhythmia may result in syncope or sudden death.

Hypoglycaemic dizziness

The commonest cause of severe hypoglycaemia is in a patient on insulin for diabetes who has either failed to eat an adequate amount or taken too much insulin. The symptoms start with a feeling of hunger followed by a cold sweat and feelings of light-headedness. Behaviour can be impaired and finally coma can ensue. Treatment is the administration of glucose, either by mouth if the patient is awake enough, or intravenously. Glucagon can be used to mobilize the patient's own glucose from glycogen stores.

Patients who have had gastric surgery can get hypoglycaemia from altered handling of food in the gut. On eating, a carbohydrate load rapidly arrives in the small bowel, resulting in a rapid rise in blood glucose. This results in a large secretion of insulin in response. If there is too much insulin secreted this may result in hypoglycaemia about 1.5–3 hours after the meal.

Alcoholics who do not eat are in danger of hypoglycaemia. Ethanol in the liver reduces the conversion of NAD^+ to NADP which makes glucogenesis from lactate no longer possible. Glucose can be generated from glycogen by glycogenolysis. However, after a 24-hour fast, glycogen stores are exhausted and severe hypoglycaemia can ensue. In severe liver disease hypoglycaemia can result from impaired glucose production.

Islet cell tumours called insulinomas are rare (incidence 4 per million), but they are the commonest cause of hypoglycaemia in non-diabetics admitted for investigation of hypoglycaemic attacks. They are associated with multiple endocrine neoplasia. Patients may be drowsy on wakening which is relieved by food or a sugary drink. Other presentations include paraesthesiae, diplopia, faintness, light-headedness, and seizures. A simple screening test is an overnight fasting glucose and plasma insulin level.

Psychogenic dizziness

Anxiety states, phobias and panic attacks are associated with a feeling of light-headedness which is often described by the patient as dizziness. Many of these symptoms are due to hyperventilation syndrome, which is discussed in detail in Chapter 6.

There remains a group of patients with various anxiety states in whom no physiological mechanism for their dizziness can be identified. In time-honoured fashion these patients are labelled functional. There is little to do apart from provide reassurance and avoid giving long-term vestibular sedatives.

Drug-induced dizziness

As most medical students are aware, some drugs can induce dizziness. Ethanol for example can produce dizziness due to its toxic effects on the cerebellum, resulting in disequilibrium. In addition, the specific gravity of ethanol can also induce a true vertigo by setting up currents in the semicircular canals.

Antiepileptic drugs such as phenytoin and carbamazepine at toxic levels produce dizziness through disequilibrium as a result of their effect on the cerebellum. Tranquillizers can also induce unsteadiness especially in the elderly who may already have impairment of proprioception and vision.

Disequilibrium

Disequilibrium is interpreted by many patients as dizziness. In older patients multiple sensory failure may contribute to this problem. Loss of proprioceptive sensation from the feet, visual impairment, and labyrinthine disease or damage to the integration of these inputs through cerebrovascular disease results in instability. Each individual aspect of the disorder needs to be addressed, but the effect of drugs such as benzodiazepines may be the most remedial factor. Physiotherapy training in safe walking and confidence building may also play an important role in treatment.

MCQs for Chapter 4

The MCQs are either true T or false F. The answers are given in Appendix 3. Negatively mark your answers; a point for a correct answer, deduct a point for an incorrect response. If you score 24 or more you pass.

1. **The following are often interpreted as dizziness by patients:**
   A Palpitation.
   B Vertigo.
   C Dyspnoea.
   D Hypotension.

2. **Drugs that commonly induce dizziness include:**
   A Prochlorperazine.
   B Carbamazepine.
   C Ethanol.
   D Paracetamol.

3. **Common causes of vertigo include:**
   A Ménière's disease.
   B Benign positional vertigo.
   C Hypoglycaemia.
   D Proprioceptive loss.

4. **Presyncope can be induced by:**
   A Tachyarrhythmia.
   B Bradyarrythmia.
   C Benign recurrent vertigo.
   D Ménière's disease.

5. **Benign positional vertigo**
   A Is caused by calcium carbonate crystals.
   B The pathology lies in the cochlea.
   C Is usually treated with surgery.
   D Can be demonstrated by the Hallpike manoeuvre.

6. **Ménière's disease**
   A Occurs in 5% of the population.
   B Is treated with salt restriction.
   C Surgery may have a role in intractable cases.
   D Causes persistent vertigo.

7. **Causes of hypoglycaemia include:**
   A Hyperosmolar diabetic coma.
   B Gastric surgery.
   C Insulinoma.
   D Alcoholism.

8. **Ethanol commonly induces dizziness because of:**
   A Its specific gravity.
   B Its effects on the spinal cord.
   C Its effects on the cortex.
   D Its effects on the cerebellum.

9. **Treatable causes of dizziness due to disequilibrium include:**
   A Diabetic peripheral neuropathy.
   B Macular degeneration.
   C Loss of confidence.
   D The effect of benzodiazepines.

10. **The vestibular system:**
    A There are two semicircular canals set at right angles.
    B The fluid in the canals is CSF.
    C The otolith informs the brain about head tilt.
    D The cupola lies in the ampulla.

5. Weakness

Objectives

In this chapter we shall explore what patients mean by 'weak'. The patterns of motor dysfunction seen in clinical practice are discussed:

- Hemiplegia
- Facial weakness
- Crossed syndrome
- 'Off legs'
- Quadriparesis   Cord
                           Muscle disease
                           Neuropathies
- Monoplegia   Upper motor neurone
                           Root
                           Nerve

What patients mean

Most patients have not undergone a medical education costing over £100 000, so their use of terminology may well be different from your own. Even those patients who are medically educated may use terms in unconventional ways, so it is always best to check what people mean. Useless, dead, paralysed, weak and even numb can all mean there was a loss of power in a limb. Patients get into particular difficulty when describing loss of dexterity. Loss of dexterity has to be distinguished from weakness and dystaxia. Frequently this cannot be done on history alone and will have to await the examination to confirm one's suspicions. Even the distinction between the sensory and motor system will not be taken as *a priori* by many patients. This is interesting as the brain shares our patient's reluctance to be so simplistic.

Hemiplegia

Hemiplegia/paresis is a common neurological presentation which is often thought as being synonymous with stroke. This is not necessarily the case. Hemi- means half, which in this case means half the body, so an arm and a leg on the same side are affected. Plegia usually means complete paralysis, while paresis denotes weakness usually of a lesser degree. So hemiplegia means weak down one side of the body. Rarely this can occur on a lower motor neurone basis, but usually the pathology is within the central nervous system (CNS), but can be anywhere from the cervical cord to the motor cortex. Large cells in the motor cortex send axons down the neuroaxis to terminate in the spinal cord on α-motor neurones. These cells are called pyramidal cells, hence pyramidal tract and 'pyramidal weakness' (Table 5.1).

Extensor weak in the upper limb
Flexors weak in the lower limb
'Clasp knife' increased spasticity
Hyper-reflexia
Babinski's sign

Table 5.1 Pyramidal weakness

Facial weakness

The presence or absence of facial weakness provides useful localizing information. Facial weakness can be of an upper motor neurone type or a lower motor neurone type. If the facial nerve or nucleus is damaged both the upper and lower face are involved. If there is unilateral upper motor neurone damage in the pyramidal tracts above the motor nucleus there will be weakness of the lower face, but much less so of the upper face, especially the brow (Fig. 5.1).

The upper face is bilaterally represented at an upper motor neurone level, which means that for an upper motor neurone lesion to produce an upper facial weakness it has to be bilateral. If the facial weakness is of the upper motor neurone type and on the same side as the hemiparesis then the lowest the lesion can be is in the upper pons where the fibres to the facial nucleus decussate. Likely sites for the lesion are above the tentorium, in the internal capsule, corona radiata or motor cortex.

When a patient presents with a hemiplegia it is important to decide if the face is involved as that will give a lower limit as to how far down the neuroaxis the pathology could be. If the face is involved the pathology has to be higher than the spinal cord. As the nucleus of the seventh nerve lies in the brain stem both upper and lower motor neurone type facial weakness can be due to pathology in the CNS. The commonest cause of an isolated lower motor neurone facial weakness is a Bell's palsy. This is an idiopathic condition, usually attributed to a virus causing swelling of the nerve prior to the stylomastoid foramen, resulting in compression of the nerve in its own canal. There is a temptation to call any facial

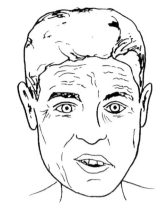

Upper motor neurone facial weakness

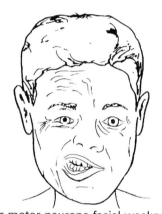

Lower motor neurone facial weakness

Fig. 5.1 Upper and lower motor neurone type facial weakness.

weakness a Bell's palsy when other pathologies have not adequately been excluded.

Crossed syndrome

A lesion on one side of the pons may well produce a lower facial weakness on that side and catch the motor fibres of the pyramidal tract on their way down from cortex to cord. These fibres have yet to decussate in the pyramids so are on the opposite side of the body to the limbs they motivate. Lesions in the pons will result in a facial weakness on the opposite side of the body to the hemiparesis; a so-called crossed syndrome (Fig. 5.2). Although this constellation of findings is rare it pinpoints the lesion to the pons on the side of the facial weakness.

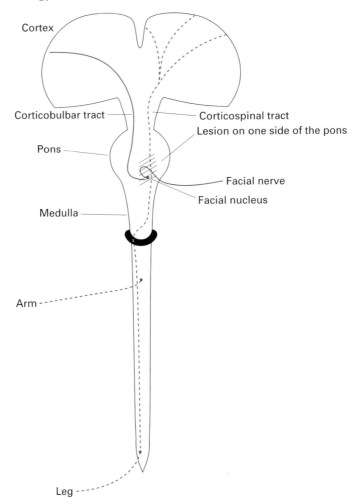

Fig. 5.2 Anatomical basis of the crossed motor syndrome.

'Off legs'

A number of factors can contribute to the common presentation of 'off legs'. It is especially common in the elderly where multiple factors act together, such as diffuse cerebrovascular disease, an element of peripheral neuropathy, compounded by a urinary tract infection may be enough to stop someone ambulating. When assessing the neurological causes for 'off legs' power has to be assessed as there may be a paraplegia (both legs weak). Both legs can be weak because of upper neurone problems, in which case it will almost certainly be cord pathology (Chapter 12).

Extremely rarely a parasagittal meningioma can result in bilateral leg weakness as an initial presentation. The cauda equina is a rare site of pathology, such as a tumour or centrally herniated disc. Usually there is bladder involvement. Both lumbosacral plexi can be involved in diabetic amyotrophy resulting in pain, wasting and proximal weakness in the legs. Rarely a pelvic tumour could involve both plexi.

Further distally peripheral neuropathies can affect both legs first, such as Guillain–Barré. Muscle disease can initially affect the proximal power muscles of the legs, making the climbing of stairs and getting up from a squat difficult.

Case history

Alan Hartshill was a 27-year old unemployed mechanic who developed a weakness of the left side of the face. This was diagnosed as Bell's palsy by his GP. A week later his right hand became clumsy and he started catching his right toe on the ground. He nearly tripped up over the pavement. He had had some tinglings in his limbs, but his predominant concern was the clumsiness in his right hand and his facial appearance.

On examination he had a lower motor neurone type facial weakness with quite profound weakness of the lower face, moderate weakness of eye closure and he could wrinkle his brow equally on both sides. There was weakness of grip in his right hand and it was clumsy. There was a mild weakness of dorsiflexion of the right foot. He was generally a bit hyper-reflexic, and his right plantar was extensor; a Babinski sign.

After further investigation he was diagnosed as having an episode of brain-stem demyelination with a plaque demonstrable on magnetic resonance imaging (MRI) in the left pons. Six months later he had an episode of optic neuritis making a diagnosis of multiple sclerosis.

Cervical spondylosis
Syringomyelia
Intrinsic cord tumour
Extrinsic tumour causing cord compression
Motor neurone disease

Table 5.2 Lower motor signs in arms, upper motor signs in the legs

Quadriparesis

If the arms are involved as well as the legs the lowest the pathology can be is in the cervical cord. If there are lower motor neurone signs such as reduced reflexes or wasting then the pathology is in the cervical cord (Table 5.2). The reflexes can be used to find the lowest point at which the pathology can be sited. The finding of a pathologically brisk reflex means that the pathology must be above that level. If the biceps jerk is very brisk, the pathology must be above C5/6. This rule is particularly useful when there are upper motor neurone signs in all four limbs. The question arises as to whether the lesion is in the high cervical cord or in the brain. The jaw jerk gives a clue in that it will be brisk in diffuse brain pathology such as cerebrovascular disease, but normal in high cervical cord compression.

Monoplegia

Single limb weakness is rarely due to an upper motor neurone lesion. Usually there is at least a hint of weakness in another limb or the face. Complete paralysis of a single limb should raise the suspicion of a non-organic diagnosis. Certain patterns of weakness in a limb will be recognizable as attributable to a nerve or root. This is addressed in a little more detail in Chapter 9. I carry 'Aids to the Examination of the Peripheral Nervous System' (Baillière Tindall, Editorial Committee of the Guarantors of Brain 1986, London) in my medical bag, as I suspect most neurologists do. There are some common patterns of weakness that are worth remembering, wrist drop suggests radial nerve pathology, clawed hand is either a C8/T1 or an ulnar nerve lesion. Weakness of opposition of the thumb and little finger is usually a median nerve problem. Foot drop, if lower motor neurone, is either L5 or common peroneal nerve.

MCQs for Chapter 5

The MCQs are either true T or false F. The answers are given in Appendix 3. Negatively mark your answers; a point for a correct answer, deduct a point for an incorrect response. If you score 24 or more you pass.

1. **Hemiparesis:**
   A Is usually lower motor neurone in origin.
   B Is commonly caused by a stroke.
   C Both arms are involved.
   D Can be due to a cortical lesion.

2. **Features of pyramidal weakness include:**
   A Flexor weakness in the upper limb.
   B Extensor weakness in the lower limb.
   C Hyper-reflexia.
   D 'Clasp-knife' spasticity.

3. **Facial weakness:**
   A Lower motor neurone type involves the brow.
   B At an upper motor neurone (UMN) level there is bilateral representation of the brow.
   C Bell's palsy is the most common form of UMN facial weakness.
   D The facial nerve exits the skull via the foramen magnum.

4. **A lesion in the pons:**
   A Will cause facial weakness on the opposite side.
   B The pyramidal tract is ipsilateral to the limbs it supplies in the pons.
   C A crossed motor syndrome suggests a lesion in the pons.
   D The pyramids are the point where the pyramidal tracts decussate.

5. **Causes of being 'off legs' include:**
   A Peripheral neuropathy.

   B Amaurosis fugax.
   C Myelopathy.
   D Carpal tunnel syndrome.

6. **Bilateral leg weakness can be due to:**
   A A parasagittal meningioma.
   B Middle cerebral artery infarction.
   C Thoracic outlet syndrome.
   D Guillain–Barré syndrome.

7. **Quadriparesis:**
   A If arms and legs are involved the lesion must be in the cervical cord.
   B The lesion is an upper motor neurone one.
   C A brisk jaw jerk implies cerebral pathology.
   D If the biceps jerk is brisk the pathology must be above C5/6.

8. **Causes of lower motor neurone signs in the arms and upper in the legs include:**
   A Motor neurone disease.
   B Guillain–Barré syndrome.
   C Syringomyelia.
   D Lumbar spondylolisthesis.

9. **Common associations include:**
   A Wrist drop – radial nerve palsy.
   B Claw hand – median nerve palsy.
   C Weakness of thumb opposition – C5 radiculopathy.
   D Foot drop – common peroneal nerve palsy.

10. **Patterns of weakness:**
    A Complete paralysis of an arm alone is suggestive of non-organic pathology.
    B Bilateral upper motor neurone leg weakness is usually due to cord pathology.
    C Bell's palsy is often due to a stroke.
    D Plegia usually denotes minor weakness.

6. Numbness

Objectives

In this chapter we shall explore the various sensory manifestations of neurological disease including:

- Numbness and paraesthesiae
- Sensory modalities
- Lhermitte's sign
- Tinel's sign
- Phalen's sign
- Hyperventilation syndrome
- Dysaesthesiae
- Causalgia
- Thalamic syndrome

Basic science – pain transmission

Numbness and pins and needles

When a patient says they are numb they may mean they are in psychological shock, have lost function in a body part or have a loss of sensation. Most patients have had experience of having local anaesthetic at the dentist or have slept on an arm causing them to wake with a numb hand. Such experiences can be used as a point of reference from which they can describe their sensory symptoms. Paraesthesiae causes less of a descriptive problem than loss of sensation as 'pins and needles' is a ubiquitous experience.

The distribution of the sensory loss or disturbance gives important clues as to the diagnosis (Fig. 6.1). Paraesthesiae in the fingers and toes could be due to a peripheral neuropathy, hyperventilation syndrome or cervical demyelination. Hemisensory disturbance can be due to organic pathology, such as demyelination, but particularly if the left half of the body is involved often no organic pathology is demonstrable. Sensory loss below a certain level on the trunk is highly suggestive of cord pathology.

Modalities of sensation

When examining a patient different sensory modalities are tested as different systems may be affected differentially. The usual modalities tested are light touch, pin prick, cold, vibration and joint position sense. Vibration and joint position sense (proprioception) travel centrally through the posterior columns, passing up the spinal cord ipsilateral to the area they supply and only decussate in the lemnisci in the medulla (Table 6.1). These modalities are particularly affected in subacute combined degeneration of the cord (B_{12} deficiency) and tabes dorsalis (a late manifestation of syphilis).

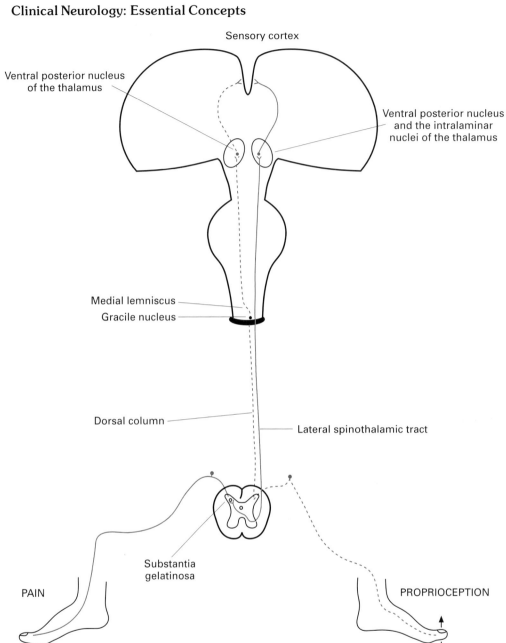

Fig. 6.1 Posterior column and spinothalamic sensory systems.

Pain (pin prick) and temperature tests are carried in the spinothalamic tracts. These modalities have decussated shortly after entering the cord. The difference between posterior column and spinothalamic is responsible for the curious differential sensory loss in the Brown–Séquard syndrome (see Chapter 12, Table 12.2). Patients are usually not aware of

Glove and stocking
Peripheral neuropathy
Cervical demyelination
Hyperventilation syndrome
Both hands
Bilateral carpal tunnel syndrome
Cervical spondylosis
Syrinx (cavitation of the central cord)
Level on trunk
Cord pathology
Hemisensory
Demyelination
Conversion disorder
Ischaemia (CVA/TIA)
Perioral
Hyperventilation syndrome
Brain-stem ischaemia

Table 6.1 Distributions of numbness

the different modalities of sensory loss, but they may report that they are unaware of where a limb is in space.

Lhermitte's sign

Lhermitte's sign is a wonderful misnomer. It was originally described by Charcot and technically is a symptom not a sign. It consists of electric shock-like feelings radiating down the back and into the limbs on flexing the neck. Patients may report it spontaneously, but usually have to be asked specifically and then invited to flex their neck and see what happens. Lhermitte's sign is highly suggestive of cervical cord pathology and is usually due to demyelination as in multiple sclerosis.

Tinel's sign

Tapping over any nerve trunk can induce paraesthesiae in that distribution. One can demonstrate this by hitting the ulnar nerve in its groove as it traverses the elbow to produce tingling in the little finger. This phenomenon is easier to demonstrate if the nerve is damaged. Tinel's sign specifically relates to tapping over the carpal tunnel

---

Case history

Alice Bentilee is a 51-year-old sponger and foot wiper who complained to her doctor of an 18-month history of tingling in the right hand. At night she would wake to find her hand numb. In addition, her life had become a misery as she was being woken from sleep by pain in the hand. She had started dropping things at work and in the kitchen and was concerned she might lose her job.

On examination there was a reduction in pin-prick sensation on the radial side of the right hand with splitting of the fourth finger so the pin was sharper on the ulnar side than on the radial. There was no demonstrable weakness in the hand. Tinel's sign was negative, but Phalen's was positive.

Electrophysiology confirmed slowing in the median nerve across the wrist. Glucose and thyroid function tests were normal. Rheumatoid factor was negative. She underwent a carpal tunnel decompression under local anaesthesia and to her great relief her symptoms disappeared.

---

producing tingling in a median nerve distribution in carpal tunnel syndrome. Although very helpful if present many of my patients with carpal tunnel syndrome do not have this present. Tinel was a French neurologist who was Chef de Clinique at the Salpêtrière in Paris and later took an active part in the French Resistance during the Second World War.

Phalen's sign

In my experience Phalen's sign is more often positive than Tinel's sign in carpal tunnel syndrome. Phalen's sign consists of extreme extension of the wrist producing paraesthesia in a median nerve distribution. It is elicited by asking the patient to put their hands together palm to palm, pointing the hands downward and then bringing the wrists as far up as possible while keeping the fingers pointing downwards. This results in forced extension at the wrists. This position is held for a couple of minutes. If positive the patient will complain of tingling in the first four fingers of the hand.

Hyperventilation syndrome

Hyperventilation is part of the physiological response to stress, which may be appropriate in the savannas of Africa when facing a lion, but is usually inappropriate in Longton, Stoke-on-Trent. It is part of the flight or fight response that involves the diversion of blood from the gastrointestinal tract to the muscles, a tachycardia and dilatation of the pupils. If hyperventilation is prolonged the CO_2, which is usually dissolved in the blood, is blown off. This results in an alkalosis of the blood. The amount of ionized calcium present in the blood is dependent on the pH of the blood and as pH increases more calcium binds to plasma proteins, predominantly albumen, resulting in less free calcium. Depolarizing membranes become unstable resulting in spontaneous firing of sensory neurones. This produces the characteristic paraesthesiae in the fingers and toes and around the mouth. If the fall in free calcium is profound motor nerves and muscles become involved resulting in tetany of the hands. The simplest first aid solution to this problem is to get the patient to rebreathe into a paper bag for a couple of minutes. This will result in carbon dioxide accumulating in the blood resulting in a return to normal pH. The bag has to be paper and not plastic as otherwise it might stick to the patient's face and the patient may suffocate.

Dysaesthesiae

As a sensory nerve fails it may start sending abnormal messages centrally. These may be interpreted as 'pins and needles' or may be more unpleasant. These unpleasant sensations are called dysaesthesiae. As a nerve recovers from loss of function there is often a period of dysaesthesiae, so disagreeable sensations can

Basic science – pain transmission

In the peripheral nervous system there are two pain systems, the fast AL fibre system and the slow C fibre system. The fast AL fibre system has free nerve endings which respond to strong mechanical pressure or extreme heat. The nerve fibres are myelinated and messages travel at 5–30 m/s. This system is responsible for the initial sensation of pain.

The slow C fibre system again has free nerve endings, but these are triggered by chemical release of histamine, bradykinin, serotonin, acetylcholine and K^+. The response is enhanced by the presence of prostaglandins (hence the modulatory effect of aspirin). They are known as polymodal nociceptors. The nerves are unmyelinated C fibres with messages travelling at 0.5–2 m/s. This system is responsible for continuous burning pain that takes a second or two to perceive.

On entry to the spinal cord pain fibres descend 1–3 segments forming part of the tract of Lissauer before synapsing in the dorsal horn. They terminate in the outermost laminae of the dorsal horn in the marginal zone (Rexed's lamina I) and the substantia gelatinosa (II). Some of the AL fibres project into lamina V. The neurotransmitters used by primarily nociceptive afferents are substance P (Arg-Pro-Lys-Pro-Gln-Gln-Phe-Phe-Gly-Leu-Met) and somatostatin. They are released centrally and peripherally where they contribute to the inflammatory response.

The second order neurones receive their input from interneurones in the substantia gelatinosa. Axons ascend in the anterolateral quadrant of the white matter. There are two main tracts, the neospinothalamic tract (lateral spinothalamic tract) and the paleospinothalamic tract (spinoreticular tract). The pathways are primarily crossed, but there is a small but significant ipsilateral tract (this may be why pain returns after successful anterolateral surgical section).

The neospinothalamic tract (lateral spinothalamic tract) is phylogenetically more modern. It arises in Rexed's lamina I and is responsible for fine localization of sharp or acute pain. It projects to the thalamus.

The paleospinothalamic tract (spinoreticular tract) arises from lamina V and responds to stimulation of Aβ, AL and C fibres, the multireceptive nociceptors. Touch causes brief stimulation and then inhibition. C fibre stimulation causes prolonged facilitation.

Most fibres synapse below the thalamus in the reticular formation, causing the effect on level of arousal. There is also an important spinotectal tract to the superior and inferior colliculi. Anterolateral fibres also end on the periaqueductal grey.

At the thalamus the neospinothalamic projects to the ventral posterior nucleus (VPN). Somatotropically arrayed tracts from the trunk and extremities arrive in the lateral part of the VPN. Trigeminal fibre tracts arrive in the medial part of the VPN. The lateral and ventral parts are referred to as the ventrobasal complex. There is somatotropic projection to S-I and S-II in the sensory cortex. Less than 10% of nerves in the ventrolateral complex respond to noxious stimuli. The most important input into this area is from the medial lemniscus. The ventrocaudal parvocellular complex area lies immediately ventral to the ventrobasal complex. It receives a major input from the neospinothalamic tract. Stimulation results in localized pain in a contralateral part of the body. In the posterior nuclear group only some cells respond, but they have large receptive fields. Paleospinothalamic projections terminate on the non-specific intralaminar nuclei and produce a slow burning pain.

be evidence of a nerve failing or recovering. These sensations can be very irksome, particularly at night. Carbamazepine and amitriptyline can have a role in their control. Opiate analgesics are not particularly effective.

Causalgia

One stage on from dysaesthesiae is causalgia where normal sensory input is misinterpreted as pain. Light touch may be unbearable. The pain from a pin prick may spread out from the original point of contact and obtain a burning quality. Causalgia is often associated with autonomic changes such as changes in skin colour. Sudeck's atrophy, in which there is demineralization of the bones of the affected limb, may result. Causalgia is not infrequently the product of relatively trivial injury. The mechanism of genesis is not fully understood, but autonomic dysfunction is important. Treatment often involves manipulations of the autonomic nervous system, such as sympathetic block.

Thalamic syndrome

This was described by Head in 1920, initially in a proportion of stroke victims with thalamic lesions. It consists of poorly localized pain of central origin. The lesion responsible for its genesis can occur anywhere along the nociceptive pathway.

MCQs for Chapter 6

The MCQs are either true T or false F. The answers are given in Appendix 3. Negatively mark your answers; a point for a correct answer, deduct a point for an incorrect response. If you score 24 or more you pass.

1. **Paraesthesiae in the fingers and toes could be due to:**
   A Cervical demyelination.
   B Hyperventilation syndrome.
   C Motor neurone disease.
   D A conus lesion.

2. **Lhermitte's sign:**
   A Was originally described by Charcot.
   B Is brought on by flexing the wrist.
   C Is a symptom not a sign.
   D Is highly suggestive of ischaemia.

3. **Sensory disturbance in both hands could be due to:**
   A Cervical spondylosis.
   B Bilateral carpal tunnel syndrome.
   C Common peroneal nerve palsies.
   D A conus lesion.

4.. **The following modalities are carried in the posterior columns:**
   A Vibration.
   B Pin prick.
   C Cold.
   D Joint position sense.

5. **Pathologies that primarily affect the posterior columns include:**
   A Diabetic neuropathy.
   B Syrinx.
   C Subacute combined degeneration of the cord.
   D Tabes dorsalis.

6. **Tinel's sign**
   A Usually refers to the ulnar nerve.
   B If positive causes tingling in the hand.
   C Can be positive in carpal tunnel syndrome.
   D Tinel was in the French Resistance.

7. **The fight and flight response involves:**
   A Breath holding.
   B Pupillary dilatation.
   C Diversion of blood to the gastrointestinal tract.
   D Tachycardia.

8. **Dysaesthesiae:**
   A May be due to a motor nerve failing.
   B May occur as a nerve recovers.
   C Is usually worse at night.
   D Opiate analgesics are frequently effective.

9. **Causalgia:**
   A Can be the product of a seemingly trivial injury.
   B Is related to autonomic dysfunction.
   C The pain has a pricking quality.
   D There is no treatment.

10. **Pain**
   A Travels in two systems in the peripheral nervous system.
   B Substance P is a natural opiate.
   C Pain reaches the cortex through the basal ganglia.
   D Many pain fibres synapse in the reticular formation.

7. Fatigue

Objectives

In this chapter we will explore the various causes of fatigue including:

- Chronic fatigue syndrome
- Postviral fatigue
- Depression
- Fatigue in neurological illness
- Sleep disorders

Basic science – sleep architecture

Fatigue

Existence is a tiring business. Surveys of the general public show that 20–40% experience fatigue lasting for more than a few weeks at a time. I would go so far as to say that the total absence of a sensation of fatigue is good evidence for impending hypomania. Fatigue is a difficult symptom to quantify, though various scales have been used for clinical trials. Excessive fatigue can be very debilitating and unlike a paralysed leg patients have nothing to show for their misfortune. Patients also feel guilty as since childhood we have all been taught not to be lazy and to experience fatigue is somehow culpable and should be under voluntary control.

Many general medical illnesses have fatigue as one of their symptoms, such as neoplasia, liver disease, and cardiac failure. This is not the place to discuss these in detail.

Chronic fatigue syndrome

There is no agreed definition of this condition, but it consists of debilitating fatigue that has persisted for more than 6 months in the absence of other identifiable physical or psychological illness. Associated features include myalgia, arthralgia, impaired concentration, poor memory, headache, sleep disturbance, low mood and paraesthesiae. In the past it was known as neurasthenia and the current lay label is myalgic encephalomyelitis (ME). 'Hard' neurological signs are absent. It often strikes previously highly motivated and productive people and lasts for years. It has occurred in outbreaks such as the Royal Free disease. Although frustrating to treat, it is not benign: the Royal Free outbreak resulted in considerable morbidity and some deaths. Because almost any symptom can coexist with chronic fatigue syndrome the diagnosis is a potential trap. Labelling any patient with fatigue as having ME is dangerous and can be an excuse for not thinking about the problems of the patient further. I have seen several patients diagnosed as having ME subsequently turn out to have MS.

Treatment of chronic fatigue syndrome consists of treating concurrent depression with antidepressants, providing sympathetic support for the patient and initiating graded exercise. This consists of undertaking a physical activity such as walking which increases gradually day by day. The increases have to be very modest. Patients often have relapses after which they need encouragement to restart their graded exercise programme. As the body does less there are physiological changes that make it more difficult to undertake exercise. Just as athletes have to build themselves up for the Olympics these patients have to build up their exercise tolerance to that of normal everyday living.

Postviral fatigue

This condition is often subsumed under the rubric of chronic fatigue syndrome/ME. Although similar mechanisms come into play in the chronic state the two can be differentiated. Many virus infections are associated with fatigue in the convalescent period. It is not unusual for patients not to be back to their normal selves for 3 weeks after influenza, or up to 6 months after Epstein–Barr virus. Many viruses can produce an encephalitis and this may not be fully recognized at the time.

It is not surprising that a number of patients are left fatigued after viral infections. If they remain inactive for long periods of time the physiological changes that accompany the chronic fatigue syndrome develop and it becomes more difficult to return to a normal lifestyle. Treatment is the same as chronic fatigue syndrome, with support, treatment of concurrent depression and graded exercise.

Depression

Depression is common and some questions directed at identifying the symptoms should be part of any neurological clerking. Enquiring about low mood, tearfulness and suicidal ideation should be standard. Occasionally, patients will be depressed while denying low mood. The features of depression are given in Table 7.1. If you do not have at least four of these symptoms you are an insensitive automaton and should consider a career in orthopaedic sur-

Sustained low mood
Loss of *joie de vivre*
Loss of libido
Feelings of worthlessness and guilt
Poor concentration
Apathy
Suicidal ideation
Tearfulness
Irritability
Fear of losing one's mind
Social impairment
Anorexia
Early morning wakening
Motor retardation
Fatigue

Table 7.1 Features of depression

gery! If you have all 15 perhaps you should talk to your doctor.

A wise paediatrician once told me that 'if you are not capable of depression, you are probably not capable of very much'. Some empathy with the misery of humanity is part of being human, but clinical depression is an illness and a cause of unnecessary suffering. The serotonin uptake inhibitors are fast and effective antidepressants. Fluoxetine has a propensity to aggravate anxiety so I prefer to use sertraline which has a slight sedative effect. The use of an antidepressant has to be introduced to the patient in a sensitive fashion as there is a social stigma attached to mental illness. The initial dosage of antidepressant may be insufficient or there may be a problem with compliance, often as a result of side effects. After the initial depression had been treated there is a danger of stopping the antidepressants too soon and allowing the patient to slip back into a depressive state. Sometimes a lower dose will suffice in keeping the patient out of depression. Social factors that have precipitated the depression need to be addressed, but the patient will be in a much better position to do this when they are no longer depressed. Depression is one of the most rewarding illnesses to treat as within a few days one can transform a patient from the depths of misery back into a normal functioning human being.

Fatigue in neurological illness

Most patients recovering from a neurological illness will experience excessive fatigue as they have to drive their nervous systems harder to achieve the daily functions the rest of us take for granted. Multiple sclerosis is particularly associated with fatigue. The fatigue can be one of the earliest symptoms and precede any abnormality demonstrable on neurological examination. Fatigue can be one of the most disabling aspects of early MS and is resistant to treatment.

Sleep disorders

Sleep disorders are extremely common and can be subdivided into disorders of initiation and maintenance of sleep, disorders of excessive somnolence, disorders of sleep–wake schedules and dysfunction associated with sleep.

Insomnia

Insomnia is a common problem and because of the misery it induces deserves more than the reflex prescribing of a hypnotic. Causes of insomnia are given in Table 7.2. The most common are depression, anxiety and drug misuse (caffeine and ethanol). Caffeine, if taken in the evening, acts as a stimulant preventing sleep. Alcohol, while having a hypnotic effect initially, as the night progresses alcohol withdrawal and its associated restlessness occurs. The wonderful term of inadequate sleep hygiene has been coined to describe those behaviours which are likely to have an adverse effect on sleep, such as daytime napping or engaging in exciting or emotionally upsetting activities too close to bedtime.

Frequently poor sleep has become a learnt behaviour with fear of insomnia resulting in increased arousal on going to bed, which in turn produces the insomnia. This can be addressed with the behavioural technique of stimulus control therapy (Table 7.3).

Depression – early morning wakening
Anxiety – difficult initiating sleep
Poor sleep hygiene – drug misuse (e.g. caffeine, ethanol)
Circadian rhythm change
  Jet lag
  Shift work
General medical conditions (e.g. rheumatoid arthritis)
Neurological conditions (e.g. Parkinson's disease)
Sleep apnoea
Learnt behaviour
Idiopathic

Table 7.2 Causes of insomnia.

Go to bed only when sleepy
Use bed only for sleeping and sexual relations
Get up and leave bedroom if not asleep in 15 minutes
Do not lie awake in bed, get up and do a non-stimulating activity
Have a fixed waking up time
No daytime napping

Table 7.3 Stimulus control therapy

Many patients complain that they do not sleep at all when polysomnography reveals they are getting a normal amount of sleep. This is the sleep misinterpretation syndrome. A sleep log can be very helpful in identifying exactly how much sleep someone is getting.

Narcolepsy

This condition occurs with a prevalence of between 2 and 7 per 1000. It is due to an intrusion of rapid eye movement (REM) sleep phenomenon into wakefulness. Onset is between childhood and mid fifties and the condition is characterized by excessive sleepiness (narcolepsy), cataplexy, sleep paralysis and hypnogogic hallucinations. *Cataplexy* is the sudden loss of tone and power in all muscles often in response to emotional stimuli. *Sleep paralysis* is the phenomenon of wakening, but finding that all the muscles remain paralysed. *Hypnogogic hallucinations* are vivid mental images, usually visual occurring on going to sleep.

The diagnosis can be difficult as any of these phenomena can be part of normal experience.

Case history

Mrs Longton is a 32-year-old right-handed homemaker who presented with increasing fatigue and sleepiness. Ever since adolescence she had had a tendency to sleep at the drop of a hat. In recent years this propensity had become more marked. She would fall asleep during the day whenever she was not fully engaged. She had even fallen asleep when friends had been invited round for coffee. She was concerned that she might fall asleep while driving. On direct questioning she admitted to cataplexy and a couple of episodes of sleep paralysis, but no hypnogogic hallucinations. On examination she was a slightly obese woman with a normal examination. She had the DR2 HLA haplotype. A diagnosis of narcolepsy was made and she was given slegiline for its stimulant properties. This was ineffective so she was tried on dexamphetamine 5 mg three times a day. On review 2 months later she was a different woman. She bounced into the consultation room. She had lost a stone in weight and reported that not only did she not sleep during the day, but she was bursting with energy. She had difficulty sleeping at night and her new assertive self had had an adverse effect on her relationship with her husband. She was on a short fuse and intolerant of her children, hitting them on one occasion. The dose of amphetamine was reduced and she had to contend with some daytime somnolence, but slept at night and was less uptight.

Subsequently the cataplexy became more of a problem and she was started on clomipramine. She became more drowsy during the day and the dose of dexamphetamine had to be cautiously increased.

Approaching 100% of patients with narcolepsy have HLA DR2 haplotype, however so do 26% of the normal population. The defining investigation is the multiple sleep latency test where the time to the onset of REM sleep is assessed by an EEG a number of times throughout a day. Patients with narcolepsy go into REM very rapidly at the onset of sleep. Treatment of the narcolepsy is with stimulants, such as dexamphetamine, while clomipramine is effective for cataplexy.

Recurrent hypersomnia

Recurrent hypersomnia occurs in the Kleine–Levin syndrome. This is most commonly seen in adolescent males and is presumed to be due to a developmental disorder in the sleep centre. It consists of excessive sleeping of between 18 and 24 hours a day and may be associated with hyperphagia and a lack of sexual inhibition. It usually spontaneously resolves.

Idiopathic hypersomnia

Idiopathic hypersomnia can occur in association with prolonged NREM sleep and is considered an NREM version of narcolepsy by some authors. Excessive sleepiness can occur following head injuries.

Sleep apnoea

The symptoms that should alert a clinician to the possibility of sleep apnoea are snoring (obstructive sleep apnoea), confusion and drowsiness on wakening, morning headache and impotence. Sleep apnoea can be either central, obstructive or mixed. Central sleep apnoea is caused by neurological problems affecting central drive, such as tumours, infarcts or demyelination impinging on the brain-stem respiratory centres. Ondine's curse is the worst case where the patients only breathe while they are awake. Obstructive sleep apnoea is due to a failure to maintain an open airway and is often due to obesity, but muscle diseases can also cause it. Obstructive sleep apnoea can be treated with weight reduction. Other options include trachiostomy or nasal nocturnal ventilation.

Sleep deprivation

Most junior hospital doctors will be familiar with this syndrome of emotional lability, inattentiveness in monotonous tasks, irritability and even mild paranoia. In addition, on the nights not on call REM rebound occurs, which consists of intrusive and frightening dreaming.

Basic science – sleep architecture

'Till death like sleep might steal on me,' – Stanzas written in dejection, near Naples – Shelley.

Sleep is divided into rapid eye movement sleep (REM) and non-rapid eye movement sleep (NREM). REM is characterized by rapid eye movements and dreaming. Cycles of NREM and REM sleep occur every 90 or so minutes in healthy individuals during sleep.

Polysomnography records the electro-encephalogram (EEG), electro-oculogram, electromyogram (EMG) with respiratory movements and the cardiac rhythm. NREM is subdivided into stages I, II, III and IV. When the eyes are closed in an awake person the EEG shows an α-rhythm of 8–12 Hz. In stage I there is loss of the α-rhythm. In stage II k-complexes appear, predominantly on the vertexes. In stages III and IV high voltage slow waves of 2 Hz become prominent. In normal sleep at the beginning of the night there is an orderly progression through stages I–IV until the patient goes into REM about 70–90 minutes into sleep. In REM there is loss of EMG activity and atonia in all skeletal muscles except the respiratory muscles and the eye muscles. There is rapid movement of the eyes under the lids, hence the name. In REM sleep there is impaired thermoregulation, hypotension, bradycardia, increased cerebral blood flow, increased intracranial pressure, increased respiratory rate and penial erection. REM can be abolished by a lesion in the pons. In a healthy adult there are about 4–6 cycles of REM per night. Twenty per cent of sleep is spent in REM. Children sleep for 10–11 hours while adults sleep 7–8. Short sleepers are defined as those who sleep less than 6 hours per night. Monoamine oxidase inhibitors and tricyclic antidepressants dramatically reduce the amount of REM. After a period of REM deprivation there is REM rebound with vivid and occasionally disturbing dreaming.

Not only is there a circadian rhythm of sleep, but there are circadian rhythms of body temperature, growth hormone secretion and cortisol secretion. The natural sleep circadian rhythm in humans is about 25 hours, which explains why it is easier to prolong a day than shorten it. Hence jet lag is worse going west to east than east to west.

MCQs for Chapter 7

The MCQs are either true T or false F. The answers are given in Appendix 3. Negatively mark your answers; a point for a correct answer, deduct a point for an incorrect response. If you score 24 or more you pass.

1. **Fatigue is associated with:**
   A Existence.
   B Multiple sclerosis.
   C Hypomania.
   D Epstein–Barr infection.

2. **Narcolepsy:**
   A Is associated with HLA DR2.
   B Cataplexy is the phenomenon of wakening with all the muscles paralysed.
   C Hypnogogic hallucinations are usually auditory.
   D Patients with narcolepsy go into stage IV sleep rapidly.

3. **In chronic fatigue syndrome:**
   A Fatigue has to be present for more than 6 months.
   B It may be associated with myalgia.
   C It rarely strikes previously well-motivated people.
   D Treatment consists of absolute rest.

4. **Symptoms of depression include:**
   A Loss of libido.
   B Excess of energy.
   C Early morning wakening.
   D Difficulty in getting off to sleep on retiring.

5. **Neurological illnesses particularly associated with fatigue include:**
   A Carpal tunnel syndrome.
   B Causalgia.
   C Multiple sclerosis.
   D Myasthenia gravis.

6. **Causes of insomnia include:**
   A Anxiety.
   B Parkinson's disease.
   C Hydrocephalus.
   D Sleep apnoea.

7. **Symptoms of sleep apnoea include:**
   A Morning headache.
   B Chest pain.
   C Impotence.
   D Obesity.

8. **In polysomnography the following are recorded:**
   A Electroencephalogram.
   B Electromyogram.
   C Sensory evoked potentials.
   D Electroretinogram.

9. **Sleep:**
   A NREM is divided into three stages.
   B REM usually occurs immediately on retiring.
   C Skeletal muscles are stiff in REM.
   D REM can be abolished by a lesion in the pons.

10. **Symptoms of sleep deprivation include:**
    A Emotional lability.
    B Inattentiveness.
    C Myoclonic jerks.
    D Dyspnoea.

8. Conversion disorders

Objectives

In this chapter we will explore the various manifestations and the management of hysteria including:

- History
- Examination   Sensory
                 Motor
                 Visual
                 Coma
- Management

Conversion disorders (hysteria)

'The diagnosis of "hysteria" is a disguise for ignorance and a fertile source of clinical error. It is in fact not only a delusion but a snare' (Eliot Slater, 1965). A diagnosis of conversion disorder puts the clinician's skills to their greatest test. The manifestations of organic disease are protean and capricious. The variety and sophistication of psychiatric presentations are legendary. The history of medicine is scattered with disorders which were at one time considered psychological, but are now appreciated to be organic in origin.

Epilepsy and dystonia are two conditions that immediately come to mind. In fact it is becoming increasingly difficult to define exactly what is meant by a psychiatric disorder. There is a complex interaction between a patient's physical and psychological state. Migraine is often worsened by stress as are some types of epilepsy.

Theory

The term hysteria carries with it certain unhelpful misogynistic resonances. The name hysteria implies that the problem arises from the womb. One might consider such notions to have been confined to the dustbin of history; however, I met a patient who had had her hysterectomy for 'nerves'. What is more she claimed that it had been effective! I suspect she is not an isolated case.

Charcot (1825–93) recognized that the disorder occurred in men as well as women and was not connected with female sexual organs. He realized it had some similarities with hypnosis. Freud, in 1895, concluded that hysterics suffer mainly from reminiscences, and that these memories were of a traumatic nature and were pathological. These memories were held in the unconscious and were held there by repressing mechanisms. Since the memories could not be expressed normally they resulted in the emotional energy or effect being dammed up. The strangled effect is converted into physical symptoms. Therapy consists of abreaction whereby the emotion of the forgotten event is released. In order that the memory is traumatic enough and is not able to be handled by normal conscious processes there has to be a great deal of guilt and anxiety. One area of life where those two emotions abound is sexuality. Childhood sexual abuse and 'normal' sexual development including the Oedipal complex are fertile ground for repressed memories, which are difficult to handle. These memories

Case history

Joan Meir was a 44-year-old personal assistant who was admitted with a rapidly progressive quadriplegia. She reported always being tired, but on the evening of admission had been working late when she knew that she would not be able to walk to the bus. She called her boss back from a dinner party and by the time the general practitioner arrived she was paralysed from the neck down. On arrival at hospital her examination revealed normal cranial nerves, but a flaccid quadriplegia including trapezius, but not the sternocleidomastoids. Reflexes were preserved and there was no sensory disturbance. In addition she failed to hit her face when her hand was dropped onto it and there were occasional fluctuations of tone in her left arm and left leg. Her vital capacity was 2.65 litres. A provisional diagnosis of hysterical paralysis was made.

The following day her examination was essentially unchanged apart from very minor movements of her toes. With resuscitation equipment available 3 mg of diazepam was slowly administered intravenously until nystagmus was noted and the patient felt drowsy. The examination was repeated with encouragement, and voluntary flexion and extension of the wrist, fingers, feet and toes was demonstrated. In addition, she was able to hold her knee in a flexed position. The patient was informed that the test had demonstrated that she would recover. The following day she was back to normal and a psychiatric opinion failed to find any major underlying psychiatric illness. She was discharged and over the subsequent 2 years had no further episodes of paralysis, but had multiple minor complaints and was a 'frequent attender' at her general practitioners.

may be real or imagined. Psychoanalysis as a therapeutic tool remains controversial, but the Freudian theory of neurosis remains valid. There is often a tenacious link between the memory and the physical symptom, such as numbness from the waist down in a case of sexual guilt.

History

The history may give clues as to the non-organic nature of the problem. A previous history of conversion disorder is very suggestive, but patients with psychiatric histories do develop physical problems. Each presentation has to be evaluated on its own merits. The history of the evolution of the problem may be atypical for organic illness. There may have been a particular psychosocial stresser, though often one is not identified. Stress *per se* is ubiquitous and is no pointer to non-organic illness. La belle indifference is also unreliable. Patients often fail to react in the expected fashion to catastrophic physical illness. The lack of emotional response may well be an affective (emotional) paralysis or numbness that allows the patient to cope with the immediate situation. Women are more likely than men to suffer from conversion disorders, but it is not infrequent in men.

Examination

Unfortunately, while one can conclude with some certainty that elements of the examination are 'functional' in origin, one can never be certain that there is not an organic disorder underlying the elaborated symptom. Frequently, patients who are subsequently diagnosed as having MS have had a psychiatric diagnosis. This is not completely attributable to the incompetence and callousness of the medical profession. As patients fail to get, in their eyes, an adequate response to their symptoms there must be a tendency for elaboration to occur. There are certain pointers in the examination that suggest a degree of elaboration (Table 8.1). The moment an organic physical sign is demonstrated, such as Babinski's response, there has to be an underlying organic problem. It is the prudent physician's duty to err on the side of making a physical diagnosis.

Sensory examination
Splitting of the midline
Non-anatomical sensory loss
Complete loss of all modalities
Motor examination
Fluctuations in power
Holding 'paralysed' limbs against gravity
Standing on 'paralysed' legs
Sitting up despite not being able to bend legs
Visual system
Tunnel vs funnel vision
Visual acuity not following psychophysical laws
Behaviour not matching visual loss
Coma of functional origin
Holding the eyes tight shut
Responding to vibration on the eye lashes

Table 8.1 Pointers in the physical examination to elaboration

Sensory

On the sensory examination if the change from numbness to normal sensation is exactly at the midline then there is a functional (non-organic) component. There is a bit of an overlap of sensory nerves giving a return of sensation in organic pathology short of the midline. Loss of sensation that includes the whole of a limb to where it joins to the trunk is non-anatomical and suggests functionality. Similarly complete loss of all modalities in the absence of other physical signs would be very unusual in organic pathology. However, organic sensory symptoms rarely map exactly onto the published dermatomes or cutaneous distribution of peripheral nerves.

Motor

When testing power if the velocity and nature of the task is varied and this produces a variable response in terms of power then it is unlikely to be organic in origin. Both myasthenia gravis and the Lambert Eaton myasthenic syndrome have to be borne in mind, as they both cause fluctuating power. Other suspicious aspects of the motor examination are where patients demonstrate more power when doing activities than is apparent on examination. For example if the patient can-

not move the legs, but can sit up or stand then some of the dysfunction is psychological. Hyper-reflexia can be a manifestation of upper motor neurone disorders; however, in conversion disorders the patients are in such an anxious state that hyper-reflexia is found secondary to the sympathetic drive they are experiencing.

Visual

If a patient has lost their peripheral vision their remaining visual field retains a constant angle of visual arc at different distances. If it was 30 cm in diameter at 2 m it would be 60 cm at 4 m. The area of vision should be a funnel as opposed to a tunnel. Patients who report a constant visual field at different distances are not obeying the laws of physics. The same is true with visual acuity. A patient with a visual acuity of 6/12 at 6 m should be able to read the 6/6 line at 3 m. It is incongruous for a patient with very restricted visual fields to be able to negotiate their way across a room full of obstacles without difficulty.

Coma

Non-organic coma gives the suppressed sadist in us all an excuse to come out. However, a more subtle assessment than the various methods of inducing excruciating pain are more likely to give a clearer indication of the problem. If the eyes are tightly shut then there is a volitional component. Even the most stoical patient cannot keep still if the end of a vibrating tuning fork touches their eye lashes. The other useful test is to drop the arm onto the face. If the coma is non-organic the arm will mysteriously miss the face.

Management

The most important aspect of management is to make a firm diagnosis as rapidly as possible. This will include doing all the appropriate tests to exclude as far as possible organic pathology. Everyone's confidence will be lost if after making a firm diagnosis of non-organic pathology doubts creep in and further investigations are ordered. As the diagnosis is tricky at times new developments will justify the revision of the diagnosis.

Once the diagnosis has been made it is rarely useful to challenge the patient. Telling patients they are making up their symptoms is singularly unhelpful and usually results in the patient going elsewhere where the diagnostic process will have to be repeated. One can communicate to the patient that the problem is being treated seriously, that it is not life-threatening and that it will probably get better of its own accord without spelling out exactly what is going on. Some patients cope well with being told that their symptoms are psychological or stress related, provided this is done in a sympathetic way and a way forward is proposed. Patients often need a way of returning to health, and physiotherapy and exercise programmes can be very useful. It is important that patients are encouraged to return to a normal life as rapidly as possible as illness behaviour has its own rewards, such as attention and various financial benefits. These inducements to remain ill are called secondary gain. Once the patient is fully entrenched with an electric wheel chair and adapted bungalow, mobility allowance and disability allowance it will be extremely difficult to 'cure' the hysterical paraplegia. Some patients with a religious inclination are helped by prayer and it may not be just the patient who is praying for a miracle.

Sodium amytal, a short-acting barbiturate, has been used for many years in narcoanalysis to release repressed feelings and emotions. This is a skilled activity that should only be undertaken by someone with expertise in dealing with the emotionally charged material uncovered. Amytal has also been used in narcokinesis to treat non-organic locomotor disorders without exploring the psychodynamics. Patients are given enough amytal until they are in a suggestible state and then the patient is told to move the paralysed limb. When the limb moves the patient is told that this demonstrates that the circuitry is intact and that the patient will recover in the next few days. Diazepam can be used for the same purpose.

Whatever method is used for dealing with the acute hysterical symptom there needs to be an awareness that the psychiatric issues have not been addressed. I find my psychiatric colleagues helpful in the minority of patients where there is concurrent severe psychiatric illness. Clinical psychologists have skills in managing anxiety and other maladaptive states and behaviours and such interventions are appropriate for many patients.

MCQs for Chapter 8

The MCQs are either true T or false F. The answers are given in Appendix 3. Negatively mark your answers; a point for a correct answer, deduct a point for an incorrect response. If you score 24 or more you pass.

1. **Disorders once considered psychiatric which are now known to be organic include:**
   A Parkinson's disease.
   B Dystonia.
   C Epilepsy.
   D Multiple sclerosis.

2. **The Freudian theory of hysteria holds that:**
   A Traumatic memories lie behind hysteria.
   B Memories are repressed in the unconscious.
   C These memories are always sexual.
   D Recall of memories will worsen symptoms.

3. **Reliable pointers to a functional diagnosis include:**
   A La belle indifference.
   B A history of stress.
   C Female gender.
   D A previous history of conversion disorders.

4. **Aspects of the sensory examination that suggest a non-organic diagnosis include:**
   A Splitting of the midline.
   B Loss of sensation to where the limbs join the trunk.
   C Preserved pin prick when joint position sense is lost.
   D Sensory loss in the hands but not in the feet.

5. **Aspects of the motor examination that suggest a non-organic diagnosis include:**
   A Paralysis with preservation of reflexes.
   B Proximal weakness but no distal weakness.
   C Fluctuations in power.
   D Sitting up despite not being able to bend legs.

6. **Abnormalities of vision that suggest a functional diagnosis include:**
   A Loss of colour vision with preserved acuity.
   B A visual field of 30 cm diameter at 2 and 4 m.
   C A visual acuity of 6/12 at 6 m and 6/6 at 3 m.
   D Diplopia in all directions.

7. **A non-organic coma is suggested by:**
   A The eyes being tight shut.
   B The arm missing the face when dropped onto it.
   C An extensor plantar response.
   D Twitching of the eyelids when a vibrating tuning fork touches the lids.

8. **In the management of conversion disorder:**
   A Challenging the patient with the diagnosis is useful.
   B Investigations should not be performed.
   C Physiotherapy is often useful.
   D Chronic conversion disorder is resistant to treatment due to secondary gain.

9. **Amytal:**
   A Sodium amytal is a long-acting barbiturate.
   B Narcoanalysis is the release of repressed feelings.
   C Amytal can be used to induce a suggestible state.
   D Amytal is a respiratory depressant.

10. **Concurrent psychopathology in hysterical conversion disorder:**
    A Most patients have severe psychiatric illness.
    B Psychologists can help manage anxiety states.
    C Psychosis is common following hysteria.
    D All patients need a psychiatric opinion.

Basic neuroscience

9. Neuroanatomy

Objectives

This chapter aims to set out some basic neuroanatomical concepts. Areas discussed include:

- The brain
  - Temporal lobes
  - Frontal lobes
  - Parietal lobes
  - Occipital lobes
  - Basal ganglia
  - Brain stem
  - Cerebral blood supply
- The spinal cord
- Dermatomes
- Autonomic nervous system
- Peripheral nervous system
- Neuroimaging

This is hard work, but fundamental to an understanding of the nervous system.

I hated anatomy as an undergraduate. I am sure the dismembering of a body and the rote learning of the origins and insertions of all those muscles has more to do with desensitization and the building of a professional elite than with the practice of medicine. Even then I found neuroanatomy much more interesting. It still strikes me as awesome that the brain, an object one can hold in one hand, is the seat of all feeling, intellect and passion.

As will be apparent from the preceding chapters a rudimentary grasp of neuroanatomy is essential in order to localize lesions and comprehend the impact on the individual of pathology. I have tried to concentrate on only the neuroanatomy that is of practical importance. I have started with the neocortex and during this chapter we will work our way down to the peripheral nerves. Of course anatomy cannot be fully appreciated without an understanding of function and the division between neuroanatomy and neurophysiology is arbitrary. At the end of this chapter we shall consider neuroimaging, which more than any other technical advance has revolutionized neurology.

The brain

The brain consists of a layer of cortex, which is the substrate of processing. Under this layer there are various white matter tracks which link bits of cortex with each other and link the cortex to the basal ganglia, which are a number of relay stations which control the whole show. I include the thalamus and amygdala in the term basal ganglia, though nowadays basal ganglia is usually restricted to mean the globus pallidus, caudate and putamen. The brain can be broadly divided into input and output areas, though this is a gross simplification and in most parts both aspects of processing are integral and the cortex reflects this. If you consider sterognosis, the recognition of an object from its shape, it is obvious that such an activity cannot be seen as simply a passive sensory process. Anterior to the Rolandic fissure (central sulcus) is predominantly output, while posterior is input.

There have been two classical approaches to the localization of function within the brain. There has been data generated from the positive phenomena seen in focal seizure, such as the twitching of a limb in Jacksonian epilepsy and the correlation with underlying pathology, and there has been the deduction of function from the results of lesions. Both are philosophically flawed in that one cannot deduce the function of a part of the brain from the abnormal activity seen in seizures, nor can one deduce the function of a part from the abnormal behaviour of a subject after a lesion. That these twin approaches have been so

successful in helping localize functions is due in large part to the modular organization of the brain, in that a function tends to be localized in a restricted area rather than spread all over the neocortex.

Temporal lobes

The medial aspects of the temporal lobes, especially the hippocampi, have an important role in memory. A patient (H.M.) once had the medial temporal structures removed bilaterally in an attempt to treat his epilepsy and was found to have a profound amnesia postoperatively. He remembers very little from moment to moment and his personal memories are restricted to years before his operation. In most patients the left hippocampus has a major role in verbal memory while the right hippocampus has more of a role in non-verbal memory.

The neocortical parts of the temporal lobe are involved in the decoding of sound. As one moves back up the temporal lobe on the dominant side more and more abstract information is analysed from sound, until you reach the angular gyrus at the junction of the temporal and parietal lobes where the meaning of words is abstracted from sound (Fig. 9.1).

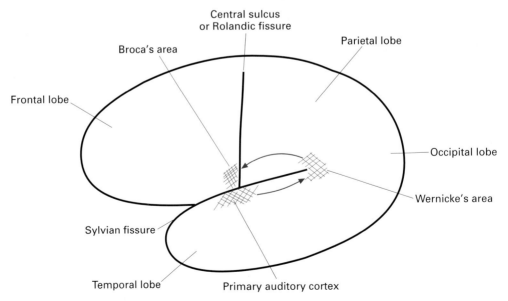

Fig. 9.1 Lateral aspect of the dominant hemisphere.

Frontal lobes

At the back of the frontal lobes lies the Rolandic fissure or central sulcus. On its banks anteriorly is the motor strip with a representation of the movements in an upside down homunculus with the legs drooping over the interhemispheric fissure. In the dominant hemisphere towards the lower end of the motor strip not far from the mouth area is Broca's area where language is constructed into speech. Anterior to the motor strip are pre-motor areas where motor commands are prepared. Anterior to this are the frontal eye fields and areas to do with attention and planning.

In 1848 a railroad foreman called Phineas Gage had an iron pole pass through his frontal lobes in a blasting accident. Surprisingly he did not die, but

'The equilibrium or balance, so to speak, between his intellectual faculties and animal propensities, seems to have been destroyed. He is fitful, irreverent, indulging at times in the grossest profanity (which was not previously his custom), manifesting but little deference for his fellows, impatient of restraint or advice when it conflicts with his desires, at times perniciously obstinate, yet capricious and vacillating, devising many plans of future operation, which are no sooner arranged than they are abandoned. In this regard his mind was radically changed, so decidedly that his friends and acquaintances said that he was "no longer Gage".' (John Harlow, one of the doctors who attended him.)

This description very well portrays the cardinal features of bilateral frontal lobe damage or disconnection. Patients have problems with planning, and they are disinhibited.

Parietal lobes

One parietal lobe is usually 'dominant' for language. In 98% of right-handed people this is the left. In left-handed people about a third have right hemisphere dominance for language, a third have left hemisphere dominance and a third have bilateral representation of language. This results in the paradoxical observation that if you are left-handed and you have a stroke you have an increased likelihood of becoming aphasic over right-handers, but you are more likely to recover.

On the dominant side Wernicke's area is localized to the angular gyrus. In this area verbal input interacts with semantics (the meaning of words). There is a white fibre tract that passes from this area to Broca's area. Also in the parietal lobe on the dominant side there resides praxis or the ability to perform complex motor activities, such as hammering a nail or turning a key. On the non-dominant side there is more emphasis on visuospatial functioning, though the dominant side is also involved in this. With the temporal lobe the parietal lobe on the non-dominant side analyses the prosodic component of speech and is involved in the insertion of prosody into output. Prosody is the inflection in speech which is so important in conveying the emotional message.

Anterior to the parietal lobe is the Rolandic fissure; on its posterior bank lies the primary sensory cortex where cutaneous and deep sensations initially arrive. This again is within a homunculus with the legs at the top. As one moves posteriorly more and more sophisticated abstractions of cutaneous sensation appear. Lesions to parietal cortex particularly damage sterognosis and graphaesthesia.

Occipital lobes

At the back of the brain lie the two occipital lobes. On their medial surfaces within the interhemispheric fissure lies the striate cortex (so named because you can see a stripe in it with the naked eye). This is V_1, or the primary visual cortex, where most of the visual input initially arrives from the lateral geniculate body. There are further topographical representations of the visual world of increasing complexity and abstraction as one moves anteriorly.

We are visual creatures. There are about a million neurones in each optic nerve and this

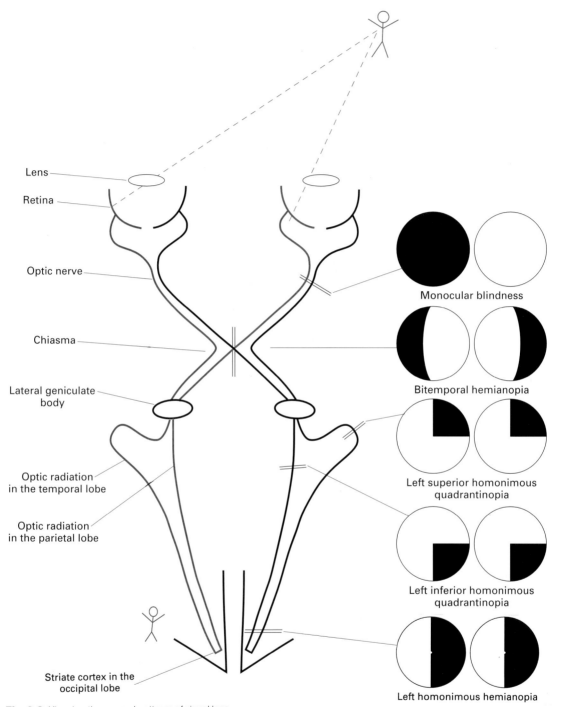

Fig. 9.2 Visual pathways and patterns of visual loss.

constitutes the largest input into the central nervous system. The types of visual loss obtained by lesions along the pathway from eye to occipital lobe are characteristic and can be used to localize the lesion (Fig. 9.2).

Basal ganglia

The term basal ganglia used to refer to the whole collection of nuclei that nestle at the base of the brain; as I mentioned previously,

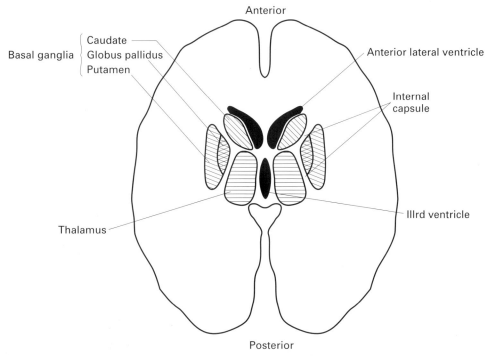

Anterior

Basal ganglia
{ Caudate
{ Globus pallidus
{ Putamen

Anterior lateral ventricle

Internal
capsule

IIIrd ventricle

Thalamus

Posterior

Fig. 9.3 Cross-section of basal ganglia and thalamus.

the term basal ganglia, currently is usually restricted to mean the globus pallidus, caudate and putamen (Fig. 9.3). The thalamus, which was included in the older definition, is the major sensory relay into neocortex, but it has a more complex role than just a relay station and important memory pathways pass through it. The lateral and medial geniculate nuclei lie in continuity with the thalamus, inferiorly and posteriorly and send their afferents to visual and auditory cortex respectively. The amygdala is part of the limbic system and has a role in memory with other temporal lobe structures. The structures now called basal ganglia (globus pallidus, caudate and putamen), are involved in the integration of motor programmes. When they are dysfunctional extrapyramidal syndromes, such as Parkinson's disease result.

Brain stem

The brain stem contains the neural substrate of basic and vegetative functions, such as respiration and the control of blood pressure. Its destruction fulfils the criteria for brain-stem

death which allows ventilators to be turned off and organs to be donated while patients are not yet dead in the traditional sense of cardioplegia.

The brain stem consists of those neural structures in the posterior fossa; that is, between the tentorium and the foramen magnum. These structures from top to bottom are the mesencephalon (midbrain), pons, medulla, with the cerebellum sitting behind the pons. The aqueduct of Sylvius goes through the mesencephalon, linking the third and fourth ventricles. This can be blocked, causing a non-communicating hydrocephalus. At the back of the mesencephalon lies the colliculi which are involved in vision and hearing.

The pons is a great meeting point of tracts. Cortical pontine fibres synapse in pontine nuclei. The pyramidal tracts pass through the pons and fibres from each cerebellum transverse the pons. It is an awesome thought that the vast majority of the output from our brains has to pass through the pons. Lesions in the anterior pons can cause the 'locked in syndrome' where the patient may only have

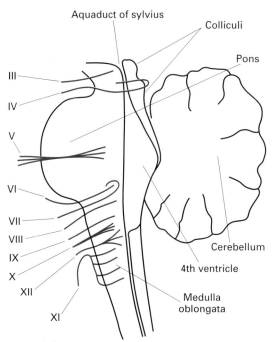

Fig. 9.4 Lateral view of the brain stem and cranial nerves.

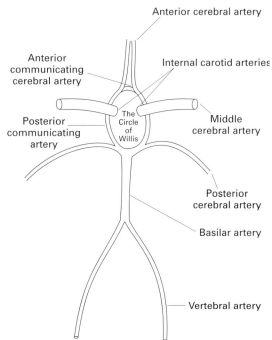

Fig. 9.5 Arteries at the base of the brain.

voluntary control over vertical eye movements, but be aware and receiving sensory input.

In the medulla lie the respiratory and cardiovascular centres. Inferiorly at the lower end the pyramidal tracts decussate.

The cerebellum consists of two hemispheres which are concerned with motor control in the limbs and a central vermis which is particularly concerned with truncal control. The cerebellum also has a role in learning complex motor acts. All but the first two cranial nerves exit from the brain stem. The third nerve nucleus is at the top of the pons, while the sixth is at the bottom (Fig. 9.4).

Cerebral blood supply

Blood reaches the brain via the internal carotid arteries and the vertebral arteries. These are known as the anterior and posterior cerebral circulations, respectively. The common carotid arteries ascend the neck and just below the angle of the jaw divide into internal and external carotid arteries. This is a common site for atheroma to form and sometimes a

bruit can be heard over a stenosis caused by the atheroma. The internal carotid then enters the skull and passes through an 's' shape known as the siphon. It passes through the cavernous sinus where a fistula between arterial and venous supplies can occur. The artery then divides into the anterior cerebral and middle cerebral arteries (Fig 9.5).

The anterior cerebral artery loops forward and upward to supply the anterior part of the frontal lobes and the superior part of the brain. The middle cerebral artery runs laterally to supply a large area of frontal, parietal and lateral temporal lobe. Strokes involving the whole of the middle cerebral artery territory are often devastating because of the large area of brain this artery supplies.

The two vertebral arteries ascend through the transverse processes of the vertebrae and enter the skull near the foramen magnum. They run up the anterior part of the medulla and fuse to form the basilar artery. This continues upwards over the pons to the mesencephalon where it divides into the two posterior cerebral arteries. The posterior cerebral arteries leave the posterior fossa and supply the occipital lobes and the medial aspect of the temporal lobes and some deep structures. The vertebral and basilar arteries give off three moderate sized arteries on each side that are called the anterior inferior cerebellar artery, the posterior inferior cerebellar artery and the superior cerebellar artery. There are also numerous perforating arteries which help supply the brain stem.

The spinal cord

At the foramen magnum the spinal cord starts and runs down to the conus at L1. Below this runs the cauda equina which consists of the lumbar and sacral nerve roots. The spinal cord has a central canal round which lies its grey matter. On the outside lie the white matter tracts which take the sensory information up to the brain and the somatic motor and autonomic commands down. The cord derives most of its blood supply from the anterior spinal artery. There are two smaller posterior spinal arteries. The blood supply of the anterior spinal artery is precarious in the upper thoracic region and it can thrombose, causing a stroke in the spinal cord.

At the back of the cord run the posterior columns. These pathways transmit vibration and joint-position sense up to the brain stem where they relay in the cuneate and gracile nuclei prior to decussating in the lemnisci. In anterior spinal artery thrombosis the posterior columns are likely to be spared, leaving preservation of vibration and joint position sense.

Pain and temperature sensation enter the cord like all sensations through the dorsal horn. They then decussate at that level or within a segment or two to travel up on the contralateral side of the cord to the area they supply (see Fig. 6.1). The spinothalamic tracts, which subserve pain and temperature sensation, travel in the anterior and lateral parts of the cord.

The corticospinal tract has almost completely decussated at the Pyramids at the bottom end of the medulla. The majority of fibres travel down in the lateral corticospinal tract to synapse on the motor neurones in the anterior grey matter at the appropriate level (Fig. 9.6). This broad separation of sensory and motor tracts gives rise to the Brown–Séquard syndrome when half the cord is transected; with power and posterior column sensation loss on one side and spinothalamic sensation lost on the other.

Dermatomes

Because the sensory system as it enters the cord is organized in dermatomes (Fig. 9.7) one

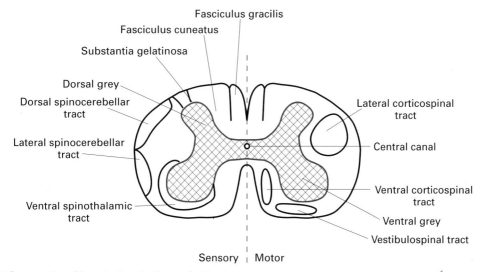

Fig. 9.6 Cross-section of the spinal cord at the cervical level.

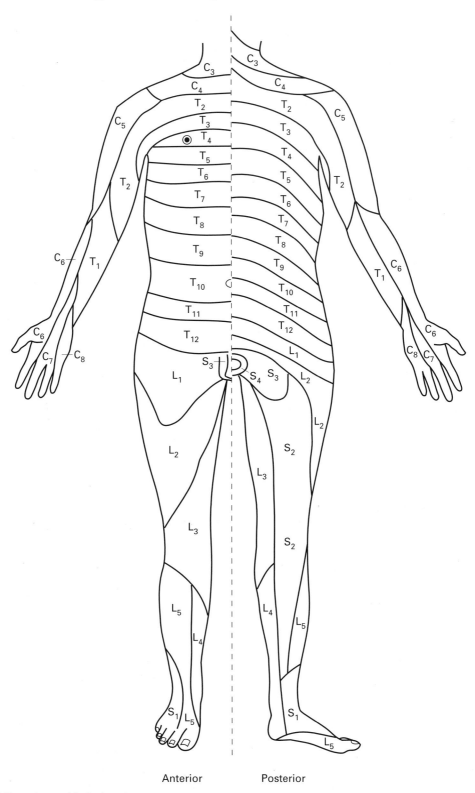

Fig. 9.7 Dermatomes of the body.

can guess at the localization of a lesion if roots or cord are affected. One of the frequently encountered errors is to presume that the lesion is at the sensory level found. Thus, if sensation is lost around the level of the umbilicus the cord lesion is at D10. First, the cord is shorter than the spinal column so a D10 sensory level will correspond to a lesion in the cord at the level of the 9th thoracic vertebrae. Second, the sensory level only tells you the lowest possible level of the lesion. It is not uncommon to have a thoracic sensory level from pathology in the cervical spine. The third trap is that the sensory level is not where sensation disappears, but where it returns to normal and this may be several segments higher. The important dermatomes to remember are:

C5	shoulder
C6	thumb
C7	middle fingers
C8	little finger
T4	nipples
T10	umbilicus
L5	big toe
S1	little toe
S5	anus

Autonomic nervous system

The autonomic nervous system is not given its due prominence in neurology text books. This may be partly because its dysfunction is not as dramatic as a hemiparesis. However, its failure can result in cardiac arrhythmia or arrest, blood pressure instability, failure to thermoregulate, loss of continence of bladder and bowel and loss of sexual function.

There are in fact two autonomic nervous systems, the sympathetic and the parasympathetic. In general, the sympathetic sets things up for 'fight' and 'flight' while the parasympathetic is more about restorative processes. Both start out in the hypothalamus and by various diverse means go down the brain stem. The parasympathetic system is also called the craniosacral autonomic nervous system because its

outflow is via the cranial nerves (III, VII, IX and X) and sacral roots. The preganglionic fibres in the parasympathetic system are long while the ganglia are situated close to the target organs and hence the postganglionic fibres are short. The sympathetic outflow is from T1 to L1. After short preganglionic nerves a chain of ganglia is formed from which long postganglionic fibres run. The differences between the two systems are presented in Table 9.1.

Both systems have myelinated preganglionic nerve fibres which is why the autonomic nervous system can be involved in demyelination neuropathies like the Guillain–Barré syndrome.

Lesions to the sympathetic system from hypothalamus, lateral brain stem and medulla, spinal cord, stellate ganglion or sympathetic fibres as they ascend initially on the carotid artery cause Horner's syndrome. This consists of ptosis (droopy eyelid), miosis (small pupil), anhydrosis (loss of sweating) and enophthalmos (never seen, but in all the books). Intrinsic lesions of the spinal cord (e.g. demyelination) cause early autonomic dysfunction with disturbances of bowel and bladder function (urgency, difficulty initiating or incontinence) and sexual dysfunction.

Peripheral nervous system

In Chapter 1, p. 2, I explained what constitutes a motor unit and the difference between upper and lower motor neurone lesions. The peripheral nervous system can be divided into root, plexus and nerve. I have already discussed the important sensory dermatomes and the roots they are associated with. There are a few important myotomes which are worth remembering. These are:

C5	Shoulder abduction
C6	Wrist extension
C7	Finger extension
C8	Finger flexion
T1	Intrinsic hand muscles
L1/2	Hip flexion

Characteristic	Sympathetic	Parasympathetic
Outflow	Predominantly thoracic	Craniosacral
Preganglionic neurone	Short	Long
Postganglionic neurone	Long	Short
Ganglionic transmission	Acetylcholine	Acetylcholine
Target organ transmission	Noradrenaline to cardiovascular	Acetylcholine
	Acetylcholine to sweat glands	
Functions	Pupillary dilation	Pupillary constriction
	Tachycardia	Bradycardia
	Cutaneous vasoconstriction	Increased intestinal peristalsis
	Intramuscular vasodilation	Evacuation of bowels and bladder
	Bronchodilation	Bronchoconstriction
	Sweating	Erection (penile and clitoral)
	Ejaculation	Lubrication (vaginal)
	Vaginal wall peristalsis	

Table 9.1

L3/4	Knee extension
L5	Dorsiflexion of the ankle
S1	Plantar flexion of the ankle

The deep tendon reflexes, which have both sensory (afferent) and motor (efferent) parts are associated with the following roots:

C5/6	Biceps
C6/7	Triceps
C5/6	Supinator
C6/7	Finger
L3/4	Knee
S1/2	Ankle

Just to add a little sport to an otherwise dull subject different books will give slightly different root values for various reflexes or movements. This is because there is some individual variability and often a number of roots make a contribution and it all depends on what is considered a significant contribution.

The brachial and lumbosacral plexi are too complex for further consideration here and I would suggest the reader consults *Aids to the Examination of the Peripheral Nervous System* (Baillière Tindall, London) when faced with a patient with a plexus lesion. A plexus lesion is suspected when the pattern of sensory and motor loss does not fit into a nerve or root pattern.

The major peripheral nerves are relatively straightforward. In the arm lesions of the radial nerve (often around the humerus) produce wrist drop and sensory loss at the base of the thumb on the dorsum of the hand (Fig. 9.8). Median nerve lesions (usually in the carpal tunnel) cause weakness of opponens pollicis and abductor pollicis brevis (Fig. 9.9). Sensory loss is on the radial half of the palm classically bisecting the fourth digit. Ulnar nerve lesions

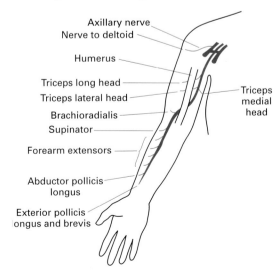

Fig. 9.8 Radial nerve course.

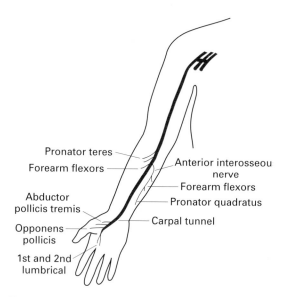

Fig. 9.9 Median nerve course.

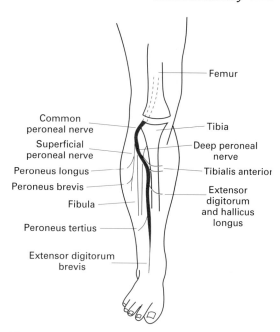

Fig. 9.11 Peroneal nerve course.

(usually at the elbow) cause weakness in flexor carpi ulnaris, the ulnar half of flexor digitorum profundis and the small hand muscles except for abductor pollicis brevis (Fig. 9.10). The sensory loss is on the palm surface of the hand on the ulnar side, bisecting the fourth finger. Femoral nerve lesions cause weakness of quadriceps femoris and hence failure to extend the knee, with sensory change over the anterior

and medial aspects of the leg centred around the knee. The common peroneal nerve passes over the head of the fibula and is a common site for compressive neuropraxis to occur (Fig. 9.11). This has to be differentiated from an L5 radiculopathy as the management and investigations are different. In a common peroneal nerve palsy there is weakness of dorsiflexion and eversion, but not inversion. In an L5 radiculopathy there is weakness of inversion as well as eversion and dorsiflexion. The sensory disturbance in an L5 radiculopathy should be more medial on the lower leg while common peroneal nerve sensory loss should be more lateral, though the sensory findings are often not clear cut.

Neuroimaging (MRI and CT)

Neuroimaging has revolutionized the practice of neurology. In the past the clinician had to wait until autopsy or craniotomy to test his/her clinical skills. The advent of rapid access to CT and MRI highlights the difficulties of localization for today's clinicians.

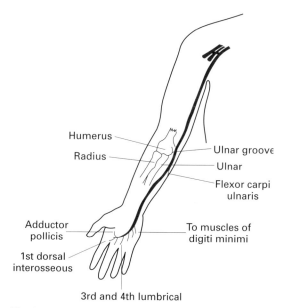

Fig. 9.10 Ulnar nerve course.

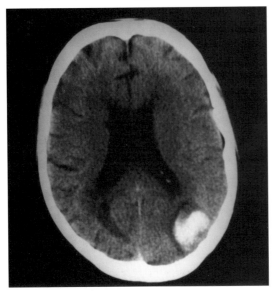

Fig. 9.12 Intracerebral haemorrhage CT at the occipito–parietal junction due to amyloid angiopathy.

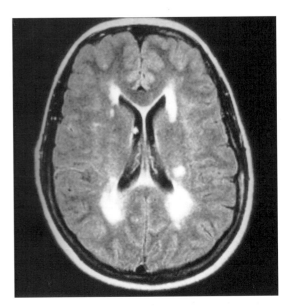

Fig. 9.13 Multiple perventricular areas of increased signal on MR (T2-weighted) in a patient with MS.

Computerized axial tomography (CT) provides an image of the density of tissues to X-rays. Blood and bone are white (dense). CSF is black and brain is grey. Differentiation between grey and white matter is not particularly easy on CT. The posterior fossa is often difficult to visualize due to artifact off the bone. Lesions obvious on MRI can be missed on CT. In addition, the dose of ionizing radiation is not insubstantial. However, it is very useful as the initial investigation of a neurological emergency. It is rapid, relatively cheap, demonstrates blood well (Fig. 9.12) and will exclude large mass lesions.

MRI is wonderful and its applications are only beginning to be exploited. It gives much better spatial resolution than CT. White and grey matter are easily differentiated. Demyelinating lesions are easily seen (Fig. 9.13). It is highly sensitive, though at times not that specific. It exploits the differences in the response of protons to magnetic fields in different tissues. By altering the parameters of the scanner different tissues can be made to produce a high signal. Like many high technology investigations it is only as useful as the person who is interpreting the films. MR angiography is being rapidly developed and functional MRI is currently still an experimental technique.

MCQs for Chapter 9

The MCQs are either true T or false F. The answers are given in Appendix 3. Negatively mark your answers; a point for a correct answer, deduct a point for an incorrect response. If you score 24 or more you pass.

1.
- **A** Anterior to the Rolandic fissure lie the input areas of the brain.
- **B** Most of the brain's processing occurs in the white matter.
- **C** Some localization of functions can be deduced from focal seizures.
- **D** Sterognosis requires motor activity.

2.
- **A** The left hippocampus is often involved in verbal memory.
- **B** The angular gyrus has a role in abstracting the meaning from words.
- **C** In the homunculus the legs are near the Sylvian fissure.
- **D** Phineas Gage had bitemporal damage.

3.
- **A** In left-handers the right hemisphere is dominant for language in 98% of cases.
- **B** Semantics are the meaning of words.
- **C** Praxis usually resides in the non-dominant hemisphere.
- **D** The prosodic component of speech is usually analysed in the right hemisphere.

4.
- **A** Cutaneous sensation initially arrives at the striate cortex.
- **B** Visual input passes through the medial geniculate body.
- **C** Each optic nerve has about a million neurones in it.
- **D** Lesions at the chiasma characteristically cause a bitemporal field loss.

5.
- **A** The thalamus is a major sensory relay into neocortex.
- **B** Dysfunction of the basal ganglia can cause extrapyramidal syndromes.
- **C** The cerebellum lies anterior to the pons.
- **D** Blockage of the aqueduct of Sylvius causes a communicating hydrocephalus.

6.
- **A** The locked-in syndrome is due to lesions of the medulla.
- **B** The vermis of the cerebellum is concerned with truncal control.
- **C** The external carotid artery supplies the anterior part of the brain.
- **D** The basilar artery is formed by the meeting of the two vertebral arteries.

7. In the spinal cord:
- **A** The spinothalamic tracts travel up the cord contralateral to the area they supply.
- **B** The majority of corticospinal tracts travel down the cord ipsilateral to the muscles they control.
- **C** The cord derives most of its blood supply from the posterior spinal artery.
- **D** In the cord the white matter lies deep to the grey matter.

8. In the autonomic nervous system:
- **A** The sympathetic nervous system is also known as the craniosacral system.
- **B** The preganglionic nerves are long in the parasympathetic system.
- **C** Penile erection is caused by activation of the parasympathetic system.
- **D** Diplopia is a feature of Horner's syndrome.

9. In the peripheral nervous system:
- **A** The sensory supply around the umbilicus is via the D10 root.
- **B** The sensory supply of the big toe is via the S1 root.
- **C** Carpal tunnel syndrome involves compression of the ulnar nerve.
- **D** Median nerve damage can cause numbness of the radial side of the fourth digit.

10.
- **A** An L5 radiculopathy characteristically causes weakness of inversion.
- **B** The knee jerk is associated with L3/4 roots.
- **C** On a CT scan blood is black.
- **D** MR scanning is very specific, but not particularly sensitive.

10. Neurophysiology

Objectives

This chapter aims to introduce some basic neurophysiology. Topics covered include:

- The neuromuscular junction
- Demyelination in nerves
- Electrophysiology (EMG)
- Reflex arc
- Nystagmus
- Internuclear ophthalmoplegia
- Dysarthria and aphasia
- Evoked potentials
- Electroencephalogram (EEG)

Without understanding physiology the diseased state cannot be understood.

I do not remember actually being taught any neurophysiology while at university except for the action potential in the squid axon by some buffer who thought he should have been given a Nobel prize. I learnt my neurophysiology by reading Kandel and Schwartz's excellent book (*Principles of Neural Science*, Kandel ER, Schwartz JH. Elsevier, New York). Anyone who is serious about neurosciences should at some stage take the time and effort to read this wonderful book from cover to cover. Neurophysiology is exciting because it is the explanation of how the system works. In this chapter I have dipped into neurophysiology to illustrate some key concepts. Of course any understanding of pathophysiology requires an understanding of normal physiology, so physiological processes will be alluded to throughout the book. In this chapter we start peripherally and work centrally.

The neuromuscular junction

It is a scary thought that the only way I can communicate with the universe is through the neuromuscular junction (NMJ). When the NMJ fails patients are left totally helpless and isolated. When an alpha motor neurone arrives at a muscle it branches into little twiglets which synapse with a number of muscle fibres. The neuromuscular junction therefore consists of a motor axon, a terminal bulb with a presynaptic membrane, a synaptic cleft and a postsynaptic membrane (Fig. 10.1). A wave of depolarization travels down the axon and arrives at the terminal bulb. This depolarization opens voltage-gated calcium channels which allows calcium to enter the presynaptic membrane. At active sites vesicles of neurotransmitter (usually acetylcholine) are released into the synaptic cleft. These molecules of acetylcholine diffuse across to the postsynaptic membrane where they bind with acetylcholine receptors. These receptors open channels which depolarize the muscle membrane which in turn opens calcium channels both in intracellular calcium stores and on the extracellular membrane. This allows calcium to enter the intracellular compartment. The rise in calcium triggers the actin/myosin ATPase to convert energy into movement. The acetylcholine diffuses off the receptor and is broken down by acetylcholine esterase, allowing the membrane to repolarize and the system to recover for the next impulse.

The neuromuscular junction is an all or none message transmission system. When a single vesicle of acetylcholine is released not enough receptors are activated to cause a wave of depolarization to be propagated over the muscle membrane. Under normal circumstances there is a safety factor in that many more vesicles of acetylcholine are released when a depolarizing wave arrives at the pre-synaptic membrane than is necessary to induce depolarization of the postsynaptic membrane. However, in myasthenia gravis, where antibodies have damaged the acetylcholine receptors, some neuromuscular junctions will be close to the critical amount of acetylcholine release when the first depolarization of a train arrives at the presynaptic membrane. When subsequent action potentials arrive the normal diminution in the number of quanta of acetylcholine released that occurs in a train may be enough to cause failure of transmission. This fall in the number of quanta usually does not matter as in health it is well within the safety margin. However, in myasthenia gravis it can lead to the hallmark of the disease which is fatiguability.

Demyelination in nerves

Demyelination (stripping of the myelin sheath off myelinated nerves) can occur in the CNS or PNS. Multiple sclerosis is a common

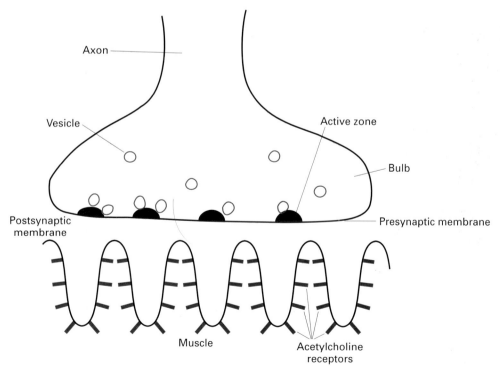

Fig. 10.1 The neuromuscular junction.

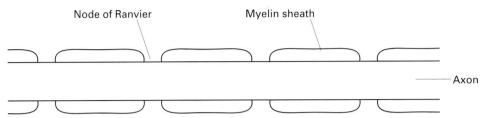

Fig. 10.2 Myelinated nerve fibre.

example of central demyelination and Guillain–Barré syndrome is a less common example of demyelination in the PNS. The myelination of nerves allows messages to be carried down axons at a faster rate. In an unmyelinated fibre each section of the nerve has to depolarize to allow the message to pass on. In a myelinated fibre depolarization only occurs at the nodes of Ranvier (Fig. 10.2). The voltage-gated sodium and potassium channels are concentrated at these points along the axon. The myelin acts as an insulator allowing electromagnetic transmission until the next node. Here the field is still strong enough to trigger the voltage-gated sodium channels. Initially I could not understand why demyelination was such a disaster for the nervous system as unmyelinated fibres work well enough albeit more slowly. However, when a Schwann cell in the PNS or oligodendrocyte in the CNS dies and exposes the nerve there are not the sodium and potassium channels present to propagate the message. In addition, as the insulation is lost the current sinks into the axon prior to the next node of Ranvier, so producing failure to transmit (conduction block). If the axon survives then later sodium and potassium channels will spread out along its length and conduction will be re-established, but it will be slower. This explains the electrophysiological hallmarks of demyelination which are slowing and conduction block.

Electrophysiology (EMG)

The major method of obtaining objective evidence about the peripheral nerves and root is via an electrophysiological examination, usually referred to slightly erroneously as EMG. EMG may be part of an electrophysiological examination, but is not its entirety. An electrophysiological examination consists of three major parts, motor nerve conduction, sensory nerve conduction and electromyography. In motor conduction studies an electrode is placed on the skin over the belly of a muscle. A reference electrode is placed on a tendon and the motor nerve to the muscle is stimulated at a supramaximal intensity some distance away. The electrical response in the muscle is called the compound muscle action potential (CMAP). Two pieces of information are obtainable from the CMAP, its size and the delay after the stimulation. By performing measurement at various points along the nerve the velocity of the myelinated fibres in the nerve can be calculated. Delays across compression points, such as the carpal tunnel or the ulnar groove can be identified. Sensory nerve conduction is performed by placing electrodes on the skin innervated by a sensory nerve. The nerve is then supramaximally stimulated at a site proximal to the recording electrode. The recorded response is the sensory nerve action potential (SNAP). SNAPs can be used to determine latency and size of response. EMG involves sampling the electrical activity of muscles by inserting a small needle electrode. Usually a muscle is electrically silent at rest, except in the vicinity of the neuromuscular junction. Fibrillations (single fascicles firing) occur in denervation and in muscle diseases such as myositis. Fibrillations (whole motor units firing spontaneously) occur predominantly in diseases of the α-motor neurone, such as motor neurone disease. The size of the responses from motor units during voluntary activity indicates the size of the motor unit. Motor units enlarge in chronic denervation.

Reflex arc

Deep tendon reflexes are an important part of neurological lore. That they cause such confusion is due to a failure to understand their basic physiology. The reflex arc consists of an afferent and an efferent part, joined by a monosynaptic connection in the spinal cord (Fig. 10.3). On tapping a tendon stretch receptors in the muscle are lengthened and a barrage of impulses passes up myelinated sensory neurones to the spinal cord. There they synapse directly onto α-motor neurones which send a barrage of impulses back down to that muscle causing it to contract. The sensory fibres themselves send off inhibitory branches and Renshaw cells within the spinal cord also form inhibitory circuits which limit the response. These inhibitory influences take longer to come into play than the monosynaptic reflex arc and so tend to limit the response

in time. If there is demyelination of the sensory side of the reflex arc such that there is slowing in some fibres there will be temporal dispersion of the response peak to tapping the tendon. As the inhibitory systems come into play shortly after the sensory input starts, if there is temporal dispersion the response will be inhibited before the peak arrives. This explains the common observation that hyporeflexia is usually due to dysfunction of the afferent arc of the reflex, so is usually a lower sensory sign. The reflex can be lost if the efferent limb of the arc is damaged, but the damage has to be extensive to be detectable.

When a part of the spinal cord is deprived of its higher (rostral) input, as in cord transection, initially there may be a diminution of the deep tendon reflexes. This is called spinal shock and is due to the loss of tonic stimulation to the α-motor neurones. So in the short term the neurones need more stimulus to fire. After a variable period (hours to days) these neurones become supersensitive and existing spinal synapses are strengthened. This then results in hyper-reflexia which is one of the major clinical findings in upper motor neurone disorders.

Nystagmus

Nystagmus refers to oscillatory movements of the eyes. Oscillopsia is the subjective experience of nystagmus. Commonly there is a fast and a slow phase of this movement (jerk nystagmus). The slow phase is the pathological process of the eyes drifting off target. The quick phase is a physiological correction. Paradoxically the direction of nystagmus is conventionally given by the fast or physiological phase. Nystagmus can be due to pathology in the semicircular canal, vestibular nerve, vestibular nuclei, brain stem, cerebellum or retina. Often the primary concern of the clinician is to differentiate central from peripheral causes. This cannot be done with certainty, but there are some pointers.

Nystagmus of a peripheral origin is often associated with severe vegetative symptoms,

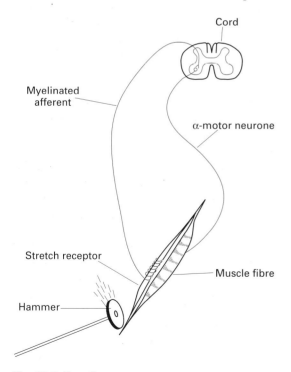

Fig. 10.3 The reflex arc.

such as nausea, vomiting, perspiration and diarrhoea. Both peripheral and central nystagmus can be precipitated by change of posture as in the Hallpike manoeuvre where the patient is rapidly moved from a sitting position to a lying position with the head over the end of the bed at an angle. Peripheral nystagmus is likely to come on after a few seconds, and is associated with nausea and fatigue on repeated testing. In addition, a particular position of the head often induces it. The commonest associated condition of this type of nystagmus is benign positional vertigo. Central nystagmus appears immediately, does not fatigue as much and the head position that induces it can be variable. Some particular types of nystagmus are particularly likely to be central; uniocular nystagmus in an abducting eye as in an internuclear ophthalmoplegia, up-beat nystagmus as in lesions of the high brain stem, or down-beat nystagmus as in lesions of the foramen magnum. Nystagmus in all directions is often due to central mechanisms failing as a result of systemic toxicity from drugs such as phenytoin. In unilateral cerebellar lesions the fast phase of the nystagmus is towards the side of the lesion whereas in vestibular damage the opposite pertains. Congenital nystagmus is present from birth and is associated with albinism and head tilt. Nystagmus can be due to macular pathology secondary to a failure of fixation. Because the macula has few rods nystagmus used to be seen in miners when mines were poorly lit.

Internuclear ophthalmoplegia

The physiology of lateral eye movements is useful to know for two reasons. First, the circuitry involves from above the pons to the lower end of the pons allowing one to check out an important part of the brain stem with simple clinical tests. Second, dysfunction of the medial longitudinal fasciculus causes an internuclear ophthalmoplegia, which is not uncommon in MS and even commoner in examinations. The circuitry is laid out in diagrammatic form in Figure 10.4. If something

or somebody on my right attracts my attention I will naturally want to foviate the object of my interest and so will want to look in that direction. The initial command to look right arises from cortical centres, however it is sent down to the lateral gaze centre in the pons which is in the paramedian pontine reticular formation (PPRF). This area tells the sixth nucleus on that side to fire, which causes the lateral rectus muscle to contract and the right eye looks to the right. I would look bizarre with one eye looking to the right and the other dead ahead, in addition I would have diplopia, so the message is passed up from the sixth nucleus across the midline in the medial longitudinal fasciculus (MLF). This is a white matter tract so not infrequently targeted in MS. Small infarcts in the pons can cause the same lesion. The MLF instructs the left third nerve nucleus to fire and the medial rectus on the left contracts, maintaining conjugate gaze. If I had a lesion of the MLF the adducting eye would fail to do so. This failure of conjugate eye movements and resultant diplopia sends the system into overdrive, resulting in the abducting eye exhibiting nystagmus to the side in which gaze is attempted. Often the lesion is partial and can only be picked up if the patient is asked to do rapid side to side saccades and it will be seen that the adducting eye lags behind the abducting. If the lesion is bilateral there will be a failure of adduction to lateral gaze. However, this can be differentiated from bilateral medial rectus palsies by getting the patient to converge. This command comes via the Edinger–Westphal nucleus and does not use the MLF, therefore convergence can be achieved. Convergence is often lost as people age so this test is only useful in younger patients.

Dysarthria and aphasia

Both dysarthria and aphasia (dysphasia) are disorders of speech, but only aphasia is a disorder of language. Dysarthria is a failure of articulation and can result from a lesion anywhere from the motor strip down to the

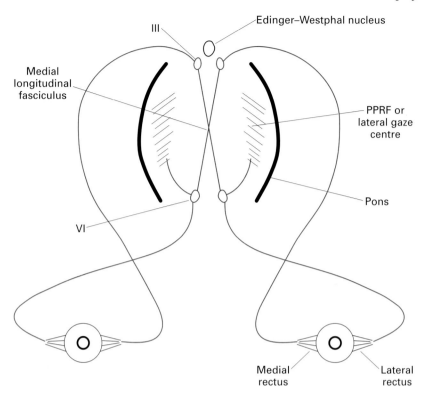

Fig. 10.4 Control of lateral eye movement.

muscles. The comprehension of language is normal, as is the language content of speech, it is just its articulation which is poor. It can be so bad that patients are left mute and is often associated with dysphagia as the same muscles are used in both activities.

Aphasia implies a brain problem. Most aphasia involve both receptive and expressive problems and both elements need assessing. There is a wonderful fairy story expounded by Norman Geschwind in the *New England Journal of Medicine* in 1971, which explains aphasia. Like most fairy stories it is not true in a literal sense, but it gives a framework from which to explain things. I shall use a modified version of it here.

Let us consider repeating the word 'Jabberwocky'. The sounds are picked up by the ear, travel up the brain stem and arrive at the auditory area in the temporal lobe (Fig. 10.5). As the message advances up the temporal lobe greater and greater degrees of abstraction occur until the message arrives at Wernicke's area at the angular gyrus which is

just in the parietal lobe. Here lies the dictionary where the semantic meaning of words can be looked up. For the task of repeating a word it is not necessary to go into semantics, the phonetic characteristic of the word 'Ja-ba-wok-ii' can be transmitted down the arcuate fasciculus to Broca's area where the word is put together again and passed to the part of the motor strip concerned with mouth, tongue and larynx movements. The word 'Jabberwocky' can then be uttered. An alternative is to go into semantics at Wernicke's area. Look up the word, realize that it is a mythical creature associated with Lewis Carol, pass the semantic message for Jabberwocky to Broca's area and again the word will be spoken. These systems break down in different ways. If semantics break down, patients can say 'tiger' instead of 'lion' for example. If phonetics are in trouble they may say 'tellingbone' for 'telephone'. These are both examples of paraphasic errors. Lesions of Wernicke's and Broca's areas form the two classical aphasic syndromes.

Wernicke's aphasia is also known as sensory

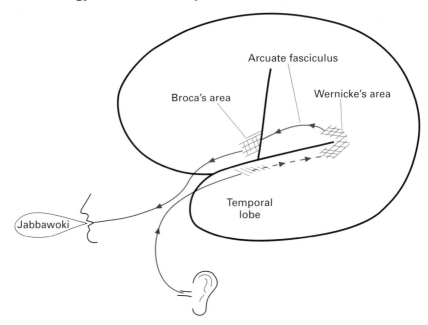

Fig. 10.5 Repetition of a word.

aphasia or receptive aphasia. The hallmark of these aphasias is that they are fluent. Many words are spoken at a normal speed; however, there are many paraphasic errors. At its worst word salad is produced. Because the dictionary is damaged comprehension is impaired, often severely. As the area is close to the occipital cortex a homonymous hemianopia is often present.

Broca's aphasia is also known as a motor or expressive aphasia. The hallmark of this type of aphasia is a lack of fluency. Few words come out, but they may be charged with meaning producing telegraphic speech, for example 'toilet go', for 'I want to go to the toilet'. The syntax, or the structure of sentences, is severely disrupted in Broca's aphasia. Thus sentences like 'No, ifs, ands, or buts about it', because they are made up of words used for syntax are very difficult for Broca's patients. In addition, patients with Broca's aphasia often have receptive problems but they are usually mild. Because of the proximity to the motor strip there is also often an associated hemiparesis.

The other common aphasia is called global aphasia and this occurs when both areas are damaged. Patients are non-fluent with severe comprehension difficulties.

The above are the commonest aphasias. There are a number of others, but they become a bit esoteric. For a wonderful read on the topic look up Geschwind's paper (*New England Journal of Medicine* 1971; **284**: 654–656). I doubt one could get away with no references on a similar paper today.

Evoked potentials

While there have been major advances in the imaging of the nervous system (MR) tests of function at present seem relatively crude; however, if used in the appropriate setting they can give valuable information with which to augment the history and examination.

Sensory and visual-evoked potentials are used to test the integrity of pathways in the CNS. They are most often used in providing additional evidence in support of a diagnosis of MS. The commonly used evoked potentials are visual-evoked potentials (VEPs), brain-stem auditory evoked potentials (BAEPs) and sensory-evoked potentials (SEPs) from the arm (median nerve) and the leg (either common peroneal or posterior tibial nerve). The principle is similar for all forms of evoked potential. A peripheral stimulus evokes a cortical electrical response. On a single event this response is lost in the noise of the background EEG. However, if the stimulus is repeated over 100 times, then the noise will cancel out, allowing the peaks and troughs of the wave form to become apparent. The usual stimulus for VEPs is a checker board of white and black squares which change from black to white and white to black (pattern reversal). As it is usually performed this test focuses on the visual system anterior to the chiasma. It is useful in a patient who has had a single episode of demyelination elsewhere in the nervous system (e.g. the spinal cord). If the VEPs show evidence of demyelination in the optic nerve (slowing and dispersion of the evoked response), then one can presume that there has been a previous episode of subclinical optic neuritis, which would confirm the diagnosis of MS.

Electroencephalogram (EEG)

The EEG involves placing an array of electrodes on the scalp and recording the potential differences observed between these electrodes. The resulting EEG is the only commonly used test of cortical function. SPECT (single photon emission computerized tomography) and PET (positron emission tomography) usually measure cerebral blood flow, though this is closely allied to cerebral function. The EEG gives two main types of useful information. It can help support a diagnosis of epilepsy and classify the type of epilepsy. The EEG gives an indication of the general functioning of the brain. In addition there are a few conditions where the EEG can be valuable diagnostically.

The EEG is the most useful test when epilepsy is considered. The only finding on the EEG that is closely associated with epilepsy is epileptiform activity which consists of spikes and waves that are clearly distinct from the background activity (Fig. 10.6). Only 2% of

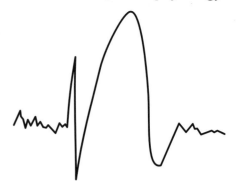

Fig. 10.6 Spike and wave discharge.

non-epileptic patients will show this abnormality. Between 50 and 90% of patients with epilepsy will show epileptiform activity of the EEG depending on the number and length of recordings undertaken. The EEG can also be used to help classify the epilepsy into generalized or focal and further subclassification. This may influence the choice of antiepileptic drugs, for example valproate for absence seizures.

The background waveforms of the EEG also give a general indication of the well being of the cortex. In a normal person there is relatively little slow wave activity, except when drowsy or asleep. When relaxed with the eyes closed normal subjects show α-rhythm which is runs of 8–12 Hz more marked occipitally. In metabolic encephalopathies (e.g. liver failure) there is a generalized slowing of the EEG and triphasic waves may appear. In dementias the EEG can remain relatively normal until the dementia becomes pronounced, but it can be useful to help differentiate from psychogenic disorders. Drugs alter the EEG, for example β activity (>8 Hz) may alert the clinician to the possibility of drug intoxication (e.g. benzodiazepines) in a comatose patient. A burst suppression pattern of activity (burst of slow waves interspersed by no activity) is a bad prognostic sign in anoxic encephalopathy. In the USA, where whole brain death is required as part of the brain death protocol, some assessment of cortical function is necessary. This is often an EEG where electrical silence or a 'flat line' EEG is required.

The EEG may be fairly specific in a couple

of clinical contexts. In herpes encephalitis there is usually temporal or frontotemporal slowing of the EEG, often with periodic sharp wave complexes over these areas. The EEG may be the earliest abnormal investigation and should alert the clinician to the need for acyclovir, if this has not already been instituted on clinical grounds. The EEG in Creutzfeld–Jakob disease may be just slowed, but often demonstrates generalized periodic sharp wave complexes, which in the appropriate clinical setting is diagnostic.

MCQs for Chapter 10

The MCQs are either true T or false F. The answers are given in Appendix 3. Negatively mark your answers; a point for a correct answer, deduct a point for an incorrect response. If you score 24 or more you pass.

1. The neuromuscular junction:
A Acetylcholine receptors are predominantly on the presynaptic membrane.
B The final trigger to muscular contraction is a rise in calcium.
C Acetylcholine esterase helps to break down acetylcholine.
D The hallmark of myasthenia gravis is post-tetanic potentiation.

2. Demyelination in nerves:
A Guillian–Barré syndrome often causes central demyelination.
B Conduction block is a feature of demyelination.
C Oligodendrocytes produce myelin in the central nervous system.
D Voltage-gated sodium channels are predominantly found at nodes of Ranvier.

3. The deep tendon reflex arc:
A The deep tendon reflex ark is polysynaptic.
B The afferent part of the reflex arc is unmyelinated.
C α-motor neurones receive inhibitory inputs from Renshaw cells.
D Hyporeflexia is often a lower sensory sign.

4. Nystagmus:
A The direction of nystagmus is named after the slow phase.
B Retinal dysfunction can cause nystagmus.
C Nystagmus originating centrally is associated with more severe vegetative symptoms than peripheral nystagmus.
D Up-beat nystagmus is common in vestibular dysfunction.

5. Eye movements:
A Activation of the sixth nucleus causes contraction of the ipsilateral medial rectus.
B The MLF (medial longitudinal fasciculus) connects the sixth and third nuclei.
C Convergence does not require an intact MLF.
D An INO (internuclear ophthalmoplegia) is often associated with nystagmus in the adducting eye.

6. Speech:
A Dysarthria is a disorder of language.
B Comprehension is usually impaired in dysphasia.
C Muscle diseases can cause dysphasias.
D Dysphagia is associated with dysarthria.

7. Aphasia:
A The entry into semantic lies in Wernicke's area.
B An example of a phonetic paraphasic error would be 'tellinbone'.
C Broca's aphasics are classically fluent.
D Patients with Wernicke's aphasia have good comprehension.

8. Evoked potentials:
A Evoked potentials are usually used to assess the peripheral nervous system.
B Pattern reversal stimuli are used in VEPs.
C A single stimulus is sufficient to produce a clear waveform.
D SEPs in the arm are usually performed by stimulating the median nerve.

9. EEG in epilepsy:
A The EEG is falsely positive in 2% of subjects without epilepsy.
B Epileptiform activity consists of spikes and waves.
C The EEG can help in the classification of seizures.
D Up to 50% of patients with epilepsy do not have epileptiform activity on the EEG.

10. EEG

A α-rhythm is at 4–6 Hz.

B A burst suppression pattern is seen in brain death.

C In herpes encephalitis the EEG abnormalities are typically found in parietal areas.

D Generalized periodic sharp wave complexes are seen in Creutzfeld–Jakob disease.

Neurological disorders

11. Disorders that affect the brain

Objectives

In this chapter you will become acquainted with:

- The epidemiology, presentation, classification and management of brain tumours
- Cerebral abscesses
- Epidural abscesses
- Meningitis due to bacteria, viruses and 'funnies'
- Viral encephalitis
- Dementias
- Encephalopathy
- Cerebral oedema
- Herniation
- Hydrocephalus
- Brain-stem death

Basic science – prions

The brain is the most important organ in the body. It is the seat of all perception, all creativity, all emotion. So as physicians our first duty is to 'save the brain'. In this chapter I will draw your attention to a number of brain-threatening pathological processes. Stroke (Chapter 15), seizures (Chapter 16), Parkinson's disease (Chapter 18) and coma (Chapter 20) are dealt with elsewhere.

Brain tumours

Most members of the public think that brain tumours are bad news, and in general they are right. The treatment of common brain tumours has not improved appreciably for the last 30 years.

There are two sorts of brain tumours, benign and malignant. Malignant in the context of the CNS does not refer to propensity to metastasize. Few brain tumours metastasize to distant sites. Malignant, in the context of brain tumours, implies invasiveness, which means they are unresectable. Benign brain tumours, such as meningiomas, have clear cut margins and can usually be totally resected.

Epidemiology

Brain tumours are less rare than one would imagine, 1% of deaths are due to intracerebral tumours and 10% of malignant neoplasms are brain tumours. The common brain tumours are gliomas (40%), metastasis (20%), meningiomas (10%), acoustic neuromas (5%) and pituitary tumours (5%) (Table 11.1).

Primary	Benign	Meningioma
		Acoustic neuroma
		Pituitary adenoma
	Malignant	Glioma astrocytoma
		Oligodendroglioma
		Ependymoma
		Lymphoma
Secondary	Lung	
	Melanoma	
	Breast	
	Bowel	
	Lymphoma	

Table 11.1 The classification of brain tumours

Presentation

Brain tumours present either by their local effects on neurological function (deafness with acoustic neuroma, or aphasia with a glioma in Wernicke's area) or through mass effect. Because the brain is enclosed in a box (the skull), if there is a mass growing in the brain, after a time the pressure in the head will start to rise. This produces headaches, which are classically worse in the mornings, accentuated by Valsalva manoeuvres (coughing, straining, vomiting) and are usually frontal or generalized. In addition, patients may complain of lethargy, slowing of cognition or drowsiness. They may develop diplopia (usually due to sixth nerve palsies) or transient blurring of vision (untreated raised intracranial pressure can lead to permanent visual loss from optic atrophy). Patients often have nausea and vomiting.

Benign brain tumours

The common benign brain tumours are meningiomas, acoustic neuromas and pituitary adenomas.

Meningiomas

Meningiomas arise from the meninges and can occur anywhere within the cranium or down the spinal column. They grow slowly and can be enormous before they present and have to have a point of contact with the meninges. This can be used to differentiate them from the gliomas which are intraparenchymal. They

enhance brightly with contrast on CT. Usually meningiomas are completely resectable and so curable. Very occasionally they are malignantly invasive. Sometimes they cannot be totally resected and re-occur, in which case radiotherapy is a second line treatment.

Acoustic neuromas

The term acoustic neuroma is a misnomer. First, it is a Schwannoma, and second it usually arises from the vestibular rather than the acoustic part of the eighth nerve. Acoustics present with unilateral sensorineural hearing loss and grow in the internal auditory meatus. Ultimately they will compress the fifth and seventh nerves and then brain-stem structures. They are the most common cerebellar-pontine angle tumour, the other common one being a meningioma. Diagnosis is made by MR scanning of the internal auditory meati. Early diagnosis leads to lower surgical complications such as severing of the facial nerve. Bilateral acoustic neuromas are pathognomonic of neurofibromatosis type 2.

Pituitary adenomas

These tumours either present as a result of their endocrinological effect (acromegaly in growth hormone secreting tumours, secondary amenorrhoea in prolactinomas), or as a result of their mass effect (e.g. bitemporal field loss). Prolactinomas respond to bromocriptine – a dopamine agonist, but the most common method of treatment is surgical by a transphenoidal hypophysectomy, provided there is not too much suprasellar extension. Postoperatively there is often transient diabetes insipidus and patients can be left permanently hypopituitary. Radiotherapy is a second line treatment. An embryological remnant left in the area of the pituitary, called a craniopharyngioma, can present in a similar way.

Malignant tumours

The common malignant tumours are gliomas, ependymomas, secondaries, and primary cerebral lymphomas.

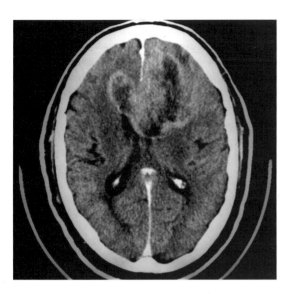

Fig. 11.1 Contrast-enhanced CT of a 'butterfly' glioma.

Gliomas

The classification of brain tumours is imperfect. Part of the problem arises from the fact that different parts of the same tumour can show different histological characteristics. Within the neuroepithelial series of tumours there are three main types of tumour, astrocytomas, oligodendrogliomas and ependymomas. Astrocytomas can be graded from 1 to 4. Grade 4 is the most malignant and a particular form of this end of the malignant range is the glioblastoma multiforme (Fig. 11.1). It is the most common primary brain tumour and constitutes 50% of all gliomas. Life expectancy is about 10 months. Treatment consists of steroids (to reduce cerebral oedema) and antiepileptic medication (if appropriate) followed by debulking where it will not cause neurological disability. CT-guided stereotactic biopsy is the usual method of making a histological diagnosis and is followed by radiotherapy. At the other end of the malignancy range a low grade astrocytoma may not progress for many years. Oligodendrogliomas tend to calcify and this is easily demonstrated on CT. These tumours are slow growing and symptoms may date back years. However, paradoxically the prognosis is not as good as once believed, median survival being 17 months.

Ependymomas

These tumours arise from the ependyma and can often present with obstructive hydrocephalus. The majority occur in children and the more malignant ones have a propensity for seeding within the subarachnoid space. Medulloblastomas and primitive neuroectodermal tumours also have a predilection for children and can seed within the subarachnoid space. The majority of these tumours are found in the cerebellum.

Secondaries

There is a baseball team in New York called the Mets. Naturally the New York Mount Sinai neurology baseball team was called the Cerebral Mets. As one would expect they had a poor prognosis and to my knowledge never won a game. The common primary tumours that metastasize to brain in order of decreasing frequency are lung, melanoma, breast, gynaecological, gastrointestinal tract and lymphoma. Some of these are frequent because their primary is common as in lung, others have a particular propensity for the brain, for example melanoma. Metastases most often present with headache, but symptoms can be very nonspecific and change in cognitive function is not uncommon. Metastases from melanoma, bronchogenic carcinoma, choriocarcinoma and renal cell carcinoma are particularly likely to present with a haemorrhage into the tumour. The primary tumour glioblastoma multiforme has a propensity to do the same. About half of the patients presenting with cerebral metastases have multiple lesions demonstrable. Treatment is with steroids and radiotherapy, but median survival is only 18 weeks. Very occasionally solitary metastases are resected.

Primary cerebral lymphoma

This used to be a rare tumour, but is becoming commoner. Part of the reason for this is that infection with HIV increases the chances of developing primary intracerebral B-cell lymphoma. Lymphoma initially responds rapidly to steroids, and difficulties in making a histological diagnosis can occur if they are started before the stereotaxic biopsy. High dose radio-

Case history

Mrs Trentham was a 73-year-old retired primary school teacher who had had a 5-month history of headaches and slight nausea. She collapsed at home and was brought to the medical assessment unit with confusion and a left hemiplegia. While awaiting a bed she had a focal seizure affecting the left hand and left side of the face. She was started on phenytoin and admitted as a stroke. A CT scan of the head showed an area of hypodensity in the right motor strip. Her hemiplegia initially improved but despite the phenytoin she continued to have focal seizures on a daily basis. She was changed over to carbamazepine and the seizures were better controlled. Physiotherapy was instituted and the hospital staff's efforts were directed at discharging the patient to a nursing home. Over the next month her condition deteriorated and her hemiplegia became denser. She was vomiting on a daily basis and lost weight. When her daughter threatened to put in a formal complaint a neurological opinion was obtained. The patient was drowsy and disoriented about location and date, had a dense left hemiplegia with visuospatial neglect to the left. There was no papilloedema. A further CT scan of the head was obtained. There was a roundish area of hypodensity surrounded by fingers of oedema spreading through the right hemisphere. The right lateral ventricle was collapsed and cerebral contents were shifted across the midline. She did not receive contrast as she was allergic to it. She was started on dexamethasone 4 mg four times a day and within 24 hours had improved cognitively. She remained with a left hemiplegia. A biopsy was performed confirming a grade 3 glioma. She underwent a course of radiotherapy, but during the course her condition further deteriorated. She was transferred to a terminal care facility where she lapsed into coma and 1 week later died.

therapy extends the median survival to 25 months. Surgery is rarely useful, unless your lymphoma is involving speech areas and as director of the CIA you have embarrassing knowledge about the Iran-Contra affair. (William Casey, director of the CIA, had surgery for his lymphoma which rendered him aphasic at the time that questions were being asked about Irangate.)

Cerebral abscesses

Cerebral abscesses act as a mass lesion. Presentation is commonly with headache, fever, drowsiness, nausea and focal neurological signs. They are the result of infection spreading into the brain from the middle ear or mastoid bone directly or through the emissary veins, or abscesses can arrive via haematogenous spread. The latter occurs in bronchiectasis or lung abscesses, or from distant sites as a result of right to left shunting in congenital heart disease. Immunocompromised individuals are also at increased risk of brain abscesses. Streptococci, bacteroides, enterobacter and *S. aureus* are the commonest pathogens. The diagnosis is made by demonstrating a ring-enhancing lesion on CT in a patient with a relatively short history. When there is a lesion in the brain that damages the blood–brain barrier, often the centre of the lesion is not well perfused, but around the periphery there is a good blood supply and a leaky barrier. If contrast material is injected this crosses the blood–brain barrier and can be seen as a white ring around the lesion. The commonest causes of this phenomenon are brain tumours and abscesses, but infarcts and resolving haematomas can occasionally give this appearance. In cases of cerebral abscess there is a peripheral leucocytosis in about 60% of cases and the ESR is elevated in 40%. Membership of an appropriate risk group aids diagnosis, but 20% of patients have no predisposing factor. Treatment usually involves surgical drainage. Care must be given to the careful handling of the aspirate as the majority of organisms are anaerobes or microaerophillic. Surgery is followed by prolonged intravenous antibiotics. Steroids and antiepileptic drugs will be necessary for some patients.

Patients with AIDS not infrequently present with ring or non-ring-enhancing lesions in the head. The most common cause is toxoplasmosis, the next most common is lymphoma. TB can also cause similar appearing lesions. It is usual to treat AIDS patients with a ring-enhancing lesion with anti-toxoplasmosis medication for an initial 3 weeks. If there is no improvement statistically lymphoma is the next most likely cause and steroids with radiotherapy may be appropriate. In general, biopsy has not been that helpful, partly because of the morbidity in patients with a limited life expectancy and partly because multiple organisms may be involved and the biopsy result could be misleading.

Epidural abscess

An epidural abscess can arise either from haematogenous spread of infection, directly from local tissues or as a complication of meningitis. It can be difficult to diagnose as the collection may not be very large in volume and imaging techniques may miss it. In the cervical spine it gives rise to a severely painful neck, fever and a rapidly progressive quadriplegia. In the head it produces headache, fever and focal neurological deficits. MR is superior to CT at imaging epidural abscess. CSF examination often demonstrates a lymphocytic pleocytosis. Treatment is by surgical drainage and appropriate antibiotics.

Meningitis

Patients with some or all of the following, headache, neck stiffness, photophobia and a positive Kernig's sign have meningeal irritation. If there is no inflammatory response in the CSF then it is called meningism and is often seen in viral infections or migraine. If there are white cells in the CSF then the patient has meningitis. Routinely, CSF is examined microscopically for organisms and how many cells can be seen per high-powered field. If there are over 1000 red cells either the lumbar puncture was traumatic or there has been a subarachnoid haemorrhage (see Chapter 15, p. 121). Up to five white cells is usually called normal, though most normal patients have only up to two lymphocytes seen. Any polymorphs should raise the possibility of bacterial meningitis. Typically, however, a bacterial meningitis will have hundreds of polymorphs present. Viral meningitis will have tens to hundreds of lymphocytes present. At the start of a viral meningitis a mixed picture of polymorphs and lymphocytes may be seen. Similar findings are found in partially treated bacterial meningitis and TB meningitis. Microscopic examination will include a routine gram stain for bacteria. Specific stains will have to be requested to look for tuberculous bacilli (red snappers). CSF is routinely cultured for the common bacterial causes of meningitis, but culture for TB has to be specifically requested. The CSF is also routinely examined biochemically for protein and glucose. The protein may be elevated in meningitis. It is particularly elevated where there is a blockage to CSF flow as in cord compression (Chapter 12, p. 96) and it can be spectacularly elevated in Guillain–Barré syndrome (Chapter 13, p. 104). The CSF glucose is most useful when compared with a blood glucose taken at the same time. The CSF glucose is less than the blood glucose, but should not be less than two-thirds of blood glucose. Low CSF glucose is seen in bacterial meningitis and sometimes in TB meningitis (Table 11.2).

Bacterial meningitis

Bacterial meningitis can be very bad, particularly when due to *Neiseria meningitidis* (the meningococcus). The mortality rate in bacterial meningitis is 10%. Patients can go from perfect health to death in a few hours. The cardinal features are headache, fever, neck stiffness and photophobia. Focal neurological deficits may be present and seizures can occur. Obtundation (clouding of consciousness) and coma are poor prognostic signs.

In meningococcal disease, in particular, a purpuric or petechial rash may be present. There are two principles of management,

	Appearance	WCC	RBC	Glucose	Xanthochromia	Gram stain	Culture
Meningism	Gin clear	0–2	<100	N	0	–	–
SAH	Pink/red	1/500 RBC	>1000	N	+	–	–
Bacterial meningitis	Cloudy	10–1000 polys	<100	Low/N	N/A	+	+
Viral meningitis	Clear/cloudy	10–100 lymphs	<100	N	N/A	–	–
TB meningitis	Clear/cloudy	Lymphs & polys	<100	Low/N	N/A	ZN+	Prolonged +

Table 11.2 A rough guide to CSF results

initiating appropriate treatment and making a diagnosis. Because of the rapidity of progression there should be no undue delay in initiating antibiotic treatment in sick patients. If there is a reasonable suspicion of bacterial meningitis the patient should be given 'best guess' antibiotics in the community prior to transfer to hospital. If possible, blood cultures should be obtained prior to administration of antibiotics. Patients who are well, but in whom a question of meningitis has arisen, require blood culture, full blood count, electrolytes and glucose. If it can be obtained rapidly a CT scan of the head should be performed to exclude an unexpected mass lesion (e.g. abscess) or generalized brain swelling. If the CT is normal and the patient is not obtunded then a lumbar puncture should be undertaken. The opening pressure should be recorded and the CSF analysed for cell count and differential on white cells, protein, glucose and culture. Antibiotics should be instituted in sick patients without waiting for the laboratory results. In adults penicillin will treat the vast majority of patients with meningococcal or pneumococcal meningitis; however, usually a cephalosporin, such as cefotaxime, is used to give broader coverage, often with ampicillin to cover lysteria. During the first month of life E. coli and group B streptococci cause up to 60% of cases. In children from 1 month to 5 years of age *Haemophilus influenzae* is the commonest organism and often requires chloramphenicol. The use of steroids in addition to antibiotics in meningitis is controversial. In children there is evidence that they lower the incidence of the commonest complication, which is deafness.

Viral meningitis

Viral meningitis is much more common than bacterial meningitis and many viral infections have an associated meningism. The difficulty arises in differentiating it from bacterial meningitis. In general, all cases of meningitis should be presumed to be bacterial and investigated appropriately. Pointers to the meningitis being viral are that the patient is still alive several days after the start of the illness without antibacterial treatment, the CSF has a lymphocytic pleocytosis, and that while uncomfortable, often with a high fever, the patients are not desperately sick. If the patient has received antibiotics prior to assessment bacterial meningitis can mimic viral meningitis and at times the only safe policy is to give a full course of best guess antibiotics. If the patient is thought to have viral meningitis treatment is symptomatic with regular paracetamol and non-steroidal anti-inflammatory drugs, and with an adequate fluid intake.

Funnies

A number of other organisms can cause a subacute meningitis. The most important of these are tubercular (TB), cryptococcus, *Borreliosis burgdorferi* (Lyme disease) and lysteria. They all present with a subacute meningitis. CSF demonstrates either a mixed or lymphocytic pleocytosis. In TB meningitis (TBM) the glucose is characteristically low and the protein high. If TB is suspected anti-tuberculous treatment may need to be initiated prior to confirmation of the diagnosis by culture. Co-infection with HIV increases the likelihood of developing TBM, cryptococcal meningitis and lysteria infection. Cryptococcal meningitis is particularly common in patients with AIDS. Its presentation can be insidious. CSF needs to be looked at with an Indian ink stain and cryptococcal antigen should be sought. It responds well to amphotericin and fluconazole treatment, but some antifungal maintenance therapy may have to be life-long if the primary immunosuppressive problem is not reversible.

Carcinoma/Lymphoma

Both carcinoma and lymphoma can cause a malignant meningitis. The neoplastic cells can seed along the meninges giving rise to raised intracranial pressure, cranial nerve and root palsies. Patients complain of headache, neck stiffness and nausea. The CSF is usually abnormal, often with a lymphocytic pleocytosis, but often repeated samples are needed to obtain positive cytology. Immunocytochemical techniques are useful in differentiating reactive lymphocytes from lymphoma cells. A gadolinium-enhanced MRI can often demonstrate meningeal enhancement. Treatment is usually unsatisfactory. Steroids and radiotherapy can be used in lymphoma. Intrathecal methotrexate is used in other malignant meningitides.

Viral encephalitis

Encephalitis is inflammation of the brain. Symptomatically it ranges from mild drowsiness, through confusional states to coma. A number of viruses can cause encephalitis, but the most important, both because it is relatively common (0.1–0.4/100 000 per year) and because it is treatable, is herpes simplex encephalitis. It presents with fever, headache, seizures and focal neurological deficits, progressing to coma. The CSF usually, though not always, shows a lymphocytosis. MRI of the brain often demonstrates increased signal in the temporal lobes. EEG is often abnormal early in the illness demonstrated by temporal slowing and epileptiform activity. PCR on CSF is potentially interesting because of its sensitivity, but the false positive and false negative

rates are unknown. In the past, brain biopsy has been used as a 'gold standard' diagnostic technique. If the diagnosis is considered the patient should be started on acyclovir 10 mg/kg 8-hourly, intravenously.

HIV can cause an encephalopathy directly and also makes patients more susceptible to other agents such as toxoplasmosis or cytomegalovirus. The latter can be treated with varying success with ganciclovir. Many patients with HIV will have subtle derangements of their cognitive function even early on in the disease, but the clinically significant AIDS dementia usually occurs later on. This can respond well for a limited period to zidovudine.

Parkinsonism

Parkinson's disease, multisystem atrophy and Steele–Richardson–Olszewski syndrome are discussed in Chapter 18.

Dementias

A dementia usually is a progressive process involving the loss of two or more cognitive functions with preserved arousal (the patient is awake). The end stage is similar to persistent vegetative state (the lights are on, but no one's home). The most common dementia is Alzheimer's disease (AD). Up to 20% of the population over the age of 80 years will suffer from dementia and 70% will have AD. AD is defined pathologically by the presence of an excess number of neurofibrillary tangles and senile plaques seen in the cortex. Plaques consist of βA_4 amyloid and tangles are made of the microtubule associated protein tau. βA_4 amyloid is derived from amyloid precursor protein whose gene is on the long arm of chromosome 21. This is of interest as patients with trisomy 21 develop a presenile dementia with the pathological hallmarks of AD. In some cases of autosomal dominant familial AD mutations to the amyloid precursor protein have been identified. Most patients with AD do not have a significant family history.

The disease often starts with memory impairments which may be difficult initially to differentiate from the normal age-related changes in memory. Later, all aspects of cognitive function are involved and social and occupational functioning become progressively impaired. The diagnosis is one of exclusion in life and can only be confirmed at autopsy. Even using strict criteria only about 70% of patients with a senile dementia of an Alzheimer's type (SDAT) will prove pathologically to have AD. See Table 11.3 for the screening tests appropriate in dementia.

Multi-infarct dementia

This is the next most common form of dementia and is currently the most preventable. It is discussed in Chapter 15.

Encephalopathy

Spongiform encephalopathies

In humans Creutzfeld–Jakob disease (CJD), Gerstmenn–Sträussler–Scheinker syndrome and Kuru are the three forms of spongiform encephalopathy recognized. They are all extraordinarily rare (incidence of CJD about 1 per million). They are caused by prions, which are altered normal proteins which induce the formation of more prions which in turn alter more normal protein. The abnormal prion protein builds up forming amyloid and disrupts membranes causing the spongiform change. These diseases have an extremely long latent period, lasting years to decades; however, the time from the first symptoms to death is usually short, being weeks to months in the case of Creutzfeld–Jakob disease. While CJD is undoubtedly transmissible in humans, as evidenced by the iatrogenic cases from pituitary derived growth hormone, many cases seem to be genetically predisposed. Diagnosis may initially be difficult. 14-3-3 protein immunoassay may be positive in CSF, but it is uncertain how sensitive this test is in early CJD. The EEG may show periodic bursts of bi- and

CT of head
Full blood count
Erythrocyte sedimentation rate (ESR)
Electrolytes (U&E)
Glucose
Thyroid function tests
B_{12} folate
Syphilis serology
[HIV]
[EEG]
Tests in square brackets are appropriate in selected cases

Table 11.3 Screening tests appropriate in dementia.

triphasic sharp complexes later in the disease. Diagnosis should be confirmed at autopsy, but because of the infectivity of the material and its resistance to normal sterilization methods special precautions have to be taken.

New variant CJD is due to contamination of the human food chain with prions from bovine spongiform encephalopathy. Currently it has only affected subjects with a genetic predisposition. It presents in young adults with psychiatric symptoms and often paraesthesiae. The EEG is not typical of CJD. The neuropathology is also distinct from CJD. Following the principle that credit should go where it is deserved I think nvCJD should be called British Spongiform Encephalopathy.

Hypoxic-ischaemic encephalopathy

This is not an uncommon outcome after cardiopulmonary resuscitation, which is why the motto 'First save the brain' is such a pertinent concept in any emergency situation. Hypoxic-ischaemic encephalopathy is also seen after near drowning, strangulation and as a complication of hypotension perioperatively or from medical causes such as MI, PE and sepsis. Complete lack of circulation to the brain for 3–5 minutes results in permanent brain damage. Often there has been a longer period of suboptimal cerebral oxygenation and perfusion. Patients usually have a diffuse encephalopathy and cerebral oedema within the first few days can result in death. Particularly resistant seizures and myoclonus can be seen. It is hazardous to make firm prognostic claims

Basic science – prions

The word prion was coined by Stanley Prusiner in 1982 to mean 'small, proteinaceous, infectious particles which resist inactivation by procedures that modify nucleic acids'. They were a revolutionary concept; a transmissible agent that caused disease which does not contain nucleic acid. The prion protein is coded on chromosome 20. In prion disease an abnormal form of the protein is formed that is protease resistant. This protein then accumulates in the brain.

In humans prions are responsible for Creutzfeld–Jakob disease (CJD), Gerstmenn–Sträussler–Scheinker syndrome, Kuru and fatal familial insomnia. CJD can be subdivided into sporadic, familial, new variant of CJD (nvCJD) and iatrogenic. The aetiology of sporadic CJD is unknown. Familial CJD, Gerstmenn–Sträussler–Scheinker syndrome and fatal familial insomnia are due to mutations in the prion gene. Iatrogenic CJD and Kuru are due to transmission and nvCJD is presumed to be attributable to contamination of the human food chain with large amounts of beef prions during the bovine spongiform encephalopathy epidemic.

within the first 24 hours, but as time goes by the likely outcome becomes more obvious. Some patients are left in the persistent vegetative state.

Metabolic encephalopathy

Almost any derangement of the milieux intérieur can cause an encephalopathy and one could conceive of the goal of homeostasis as being the maintenance of normal brain function. Hepatic encephalopathy, diabetic encephalopathy (diabetic ketoacidosis and hyperosmolar coma), hyponatraemic encephalopathy, hypercalcaemia and renal failure are the most common metabolic encephalopathies encountered. Treatment should be directed to the underlying cause where that is possible. Hepatic encephalopathy can be seen with normal liver enzyme levels in the blood in end-stage cirrhotics. Patients characteristically

have a 'liver flap' in that when they hold out their hands there is transitory loss of extension. They also have a constructional apraxia, having difficulty in constructing a five pointed star. Herniation from cerebral oedema is the major risk in acute hyponatraemic encephalopathy, but the hyponatraemia itself, as it is usually iatrogenic, rapidly and spontaneously resolves. In chronic hyponatraemia the sodium should not be allowed to rise by more than 10 mmol/l per 24 hours otherwise there is an increased risk of permanent brain damage such as central pontine myelinolysis.

Toxic encephalopathy

Most medical students have extensive experience of this condition, usually ethanol related, but occasionally precipitated by other substances. There is a vast range of chemicals that once in the blood stream alter brain function. The more common iatrogenic causes are benzodiazepines, opiates, antidepressants and, less commonly these days, barbiturates. Lithium can cause an encephalopathy associated with tremor that on occasion can be permanent. Toxic encephalopathy secondary to ingestion of drugs is the single most common cause of coma of unknown aetiology. The key to the diagnosis is an appropriate history. Carbon monoxide poisoning and heavy metal exposure are two rare but important causes of encephalopathy to be considered.

Hypertensive encephalopathy

Hypertensive encephalopathy is rare, but is not infrequently part of the differential diagnosis in patients who are encephalopathic and hypertensive. Patients who complain of headache, nausea and vomiting, are encephalopathic with papilloedema and may have seizures. They have a diastolic blood pressure of 130 mmHg or above. It is more common if the hypertension is of relatively short duration as the cerebral vasculature will not have made adaptive changes. Other causes of hypertension and encephalopathy have to be considered, such as ischaemic stroke, intracerebral haemorrhage and subarachnoid haemorrhage.

A CT scan will be required to look for evidence of these. Treatment is tricky as a sudden drop in blood pressure will produce cerebral ischaemia. The diastolic blood pressure should be brought down to 110 mmHg over several hours. The simplest way to do this is with sublingual nifedipine; however, this occasionally produces precipitous falls in blood pressure. A nitroprusside infusion has the advantage of greater control.

Cerebral oedema

Cerebral oedema is important as it is the cause of many of the symptoms patients suffer with cerebral pathology and because it produces a mass effect often resulting in herniation and death.

There are two sorts of cerebral oedema, vasogenic and cytotoxic. Somewhat paradoxically vasogenic oedema is the sort that is present around brain tumours and abscesses. The capillaries are leaky and fluid enters the parenchyma. Vasogenic oedema responds well to corticosteroids. Cytotoxic oedema occurs when brain cells die, as in a cerebral infarction. The trial data suggests that this sort of oedema does not respond to steroids and steroids are not used routinely in the management of stroke. However, from personal experience I have seen occasional cases where a patient was moribund and the administration of steroids had a close temporal relationship with an unexpected improvement.

Herniation

Herniation refers to the movement of the contents of one compartment of the brain into another compartment and is the result of pressure gradients. Raised intracranial pressure itself will not cause herniation (as in a communicating hydrocephalus). The shift of contents is dependent on a pressure gradient (Table 11.4).

A typical scenario for herniation would be a patient who has had a haemorrhage in one hemisphere (Fig. 11.2).

The haemorrhage acts as a space-occupying lesion and sets up a pressure gradient (Table 11.5). As the brain has the consistency of porridge there will be a shift of contents in response to this gradient. In the example given there will be some uncal herniation where the uncus of the temporal lobe is pressed against the brain stem. This will compress the third nerve on that side resulting in a dilating pupil on the side of the lesion. If a patient has a hemiparesis on one side and a dilating pupil on the other, one's first concern will be that they are herniating.

Occasionally the brain stem is shifted across and the third nerve is caught on the tentorium, giving a third nerve palsy on the same side as the hemiparesis. As the herniation progresses central herniation appears. This is where the supratentorial contents try to go infratentorially compressing and displacing the brain stem. This results in damage to the brain stem, both directly through compression and traction on its blood supply. If this continues brain-stem reflexes are lost and the patient becomes a potential candidate for the organ donor programme. In order to avoid this unhappy eventuality there are four simple manoeuvres available to the clinician (Table 11.6).

Mannitol is an osmotic diuretic and will suck water out of the extravascular compartment into the intravascular, dehydrating the brain a little. This will give a little more room in the intracranial box. *Steroids* reduce vasogenic oedema and may have other mechanisms of reducing intracranial pressure. *Hyperventilation* drops intra-arterial PCO_2, this produces some vasoconstriction within the skull thus reducing pressure. In addition, the patient is about to

Brain swelling
Cytotoxic oedema
Vasogenic oedema
SOL
Blood
Tumours
Abscess
Non-communicating hydrocephalus.

Table 11.4 Causes of herniation

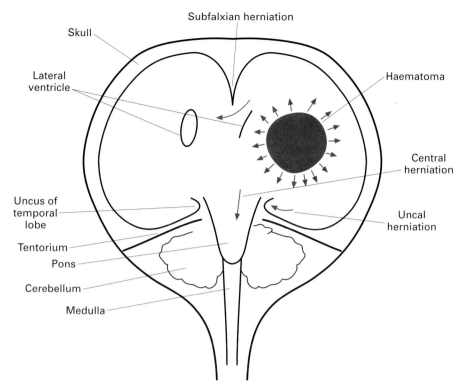

Subfalxian herniation

Skull

Lateral ventricle

Haematoma

Central herniation

Uncus of temporal lobe

Uncal herniation

Tentorium

Pons

Cerebellum

Medulla

Fig. 11.2 Coronal section of the brain herniating secondary to lobar haematoma.

Decreased level of consciousness
Nausea and vomiting
Headache
Papilloedema (unreliable and late)
Localizing signs, e.g. hemiparesis
Third nerve palsy
Loss of brain-stem reflexes

Table 11.5 Signs of incipient and on-going herniation

stop breathing anyway as the brain stem is compressed and ventilating the patient will avoid the added insult of hypoxia. The reasons for urgent CT scanning for a neurosurgically remediable lesion are self-evident.

500 ml of 20% mannitol i.v.
10 mg dexamethaspme i.v.
Intubate and hyperventilate
CT for neurosurgically remediable lesion

Table 11.6 Management of herniation

Communicating versus non-communicating hydrocephalus

This differentiation causes a great deal of confusion and is important as management of the two conditions is radically different. In *communicating hydrocephalus* there is a blockage to CSF absorption at the arachnoid villi (e.g. as a complication of meningitis or subarachnoid haemorrhage). This results in increased intracranial pressure and dilatation of the whole of the ventricular system. Patients complain of nausea and headache and may have papilloedema. However, because the CSF is in communication throughout the CNS there is no pressure gradient, hence no danger of herniation. One effective therapeutic manoeuvre would be to do a lumbar puncture as this would relieve the pressure throughout the CNS.

In *non-communicating hydrocephalus* there is a blockage to the flow of CSF from the choroid

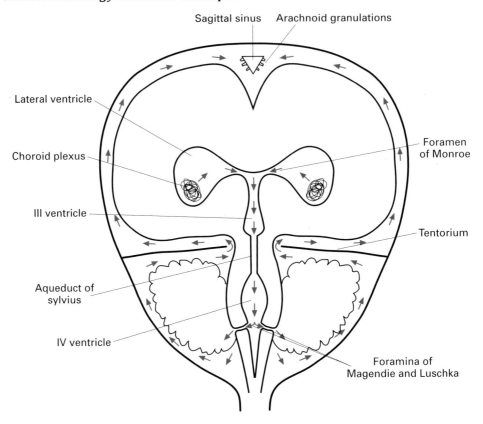

Fig. 11.3 Coronal section of the brain demonstrating the normal flow of CSF.

plexus to the arachnoid villi, usually at the aqueduct of Sylvius (Fig 11.3). This results in dilatation of the ventricular system and increased pressure proximal to the blockage. Patients will again complain of nausea and headache and may have papilloedema. However, a lumbar puncture, by lowering the pressure distal to the blockage, increases the pressure gradient and so may precipitate herniation. The treatment options are to either remove the lesion or insert an intraventricular shunt, or both. Differentiating communicating from non-communicating hydrocephalus is tricky and is usually based on a decision about the relative size of the fourth ventricle. If it is dilated then it will usually be a communicating hydrocephalus. This can be done with CT, but MRI has a number of advantages; not only does it give better anatomical resolution, particularly in the posterior

fossa, but flow voids seen within the CSF can confirm freedom of movement.

Brain-stem death (brain death)

The development of intensive care with artificial means of life support and the needs of the cadaveric organ transplantation programmes were the twin spurs to the development of the concept of brain death. It is futile, emotionally traumatic and expensive (deprives others of resources) to keep brain dead people in intensive care beds. Many organs rapidly become damaged after cessation of the circulation, hence the need for criteria other than cardioplegia for death. In the USA the concept of whole brain death developed. In the UK the concept of brain-stem death was conceived. They are usually the same, but there has been a certain amount of semantic dishonesty in some of the debate about brain death. Without a brain stem there is no future. Not only do all the vegetative functions lie there, such as the cardiovascular and respiratory centres, but the reticular activating system originates in the brain stem and without this the hemispheres will not be aroused (wake up). Usually in the catastrophic situations where brain death is being considered there has been either a bleed into the intracranial cavity or sufficient brain death and oedema to cause intracranial pressure to rise substantially. Once intracranial pressure rises sufficiently to collapse the thin-walled veins, there is no cerebral perfusion pressure and the whole brain dies.

In the UK there is a brain death protocol which should be followed religiously to avoid the possibility of misdiagnosis. Not only would an error be unfortunate for the patient concerned, but if such an error came to the attention of the media it would have disastrous consequences on the transplantation programme. The first and central requirement of the protocol is that there is a sufficient reason for brain death to have occurred; a secure diagnosis. Secondly there must be no reasons why the examination of the brain-stem reflexes should not be an accurate reflection of the health of the brain stem. This means that the protocol cannot proceed while that patient is hypothermic, sedated (e.g. barbiturates) or has neuromuscular blocking agents present, is

1. Pupillary responses to light
2. Corneal reflex
3. Oculocephalic responses to: Dolls eyes   Cold calorics
4. Gag and tracheal reflex
5. Motor responses in cranial nerves to painful stimulation of the limbs
6. No respiratory effort (with $Paco_2 > 6.65$ kPa)

Table 11.7 Brain-stem reflexes tested to ascertain brain death

metabolically abnormal (e.g. hyponatraemic) nor is there an endocrinological reason for dysfunction (hypothyroidism). The brain-stem reflexes (Table 11.7) are then tested by two senior clinicians familiar with the protocol. The examination is then repeated sometime later by the same clinicians. If the criteria of the protocol have been fulfilled and no brain-stem reflexes are present the patient is then legally dead. Life supporting techniques can then be removed or organs harvested. The time between examinations is not specified, but in general I feel it should be 12 hours, but in patients who have suffered ischaemic/hypoxic brain damage 24 hours is a safer interval. Occasionally it will be obvious that it is safe for it to be less than 12 hours. The assessment of brain death in children is more problematic and even more caution is required.

MCQs for Chapter 11

The MCQs are either true T or false F. The answers are given in Appendix 3. Negatively mark your answers; a point for a correct answer, deduct a point for an incorrect response. If you score 24 or more you pass.

1. **Benign brain tumours:**
   A Meningiomas enhance brightly with contrast on CT.
   B Acoustic neuromas present with unilateral conductive deafness.
   C Bilateral acoustic neuromas are pathognomonic of neurofibromatosis type II.
   D Pituitary adenomas cause binasal field loss.

2. **Malignant brain tumours**
   A Primary malignant brain tumours usually metastasize.
   B Prostate is a common secondary brain tumour.
   C HIV infection is associated with the development of B-cell cerebral lymphoma.
   D Glioblastoma multiforme is associated with a life expectancy of about 10 months.

3.
   A Bronchiectasis is a risk factor for cerebral abscess.
   B The ESR is inevitably elevated in cerebral abscess.
   C The most common ring-enhancing lesion in AIDS patients is toxoplasmosis.
   D The first line therapy for epidural abscess is intravenous antibiotics.

4. **In bacterial meningitis:**
   A The CSF contains hundreds of lymphocytes.
   B The CSF glucose is often less than two-thirds of blood glucose.
   C The mortality rate is about 10%.
   D During the first month of life *Neisseria meningitidis* is the most common organism.

5.
   A Bacterial meningitis is commoner than viral meningitis.
   B Cryptococcal meningitis is particularly common in AIDS.
   C In carcinomatous meningitis a gadolinium-enhanced MRI will often demonstrate meningeal enhancement.
   D In TB meningitis the glucose in the CSF is usually high and the protein low.

6. **Viral encephalitis:**
   A The treatment of choice in herpes simplex encephalitis is ganciclovir 10 mg/kg 8-hourly.
   B AIDS dementia responds to zidovudine.
   C Herpes simplex virus has a propensity for the temporal lobes.
   D Focal neurological signs make a viral encephalitis unlikely.

7. **Appropriate investigations in dementia are:**
   A CT of the head.
   B Thyroid function tests.
   C Ferritin.
   D Phytanic acid.

8. **Encephalopathies:**
   A Bovine spongiform encephalopathy is caused by prions.
   B A constructive apraxia is common in hepatic encephalopathy.
   C In chronic severe hyponatraemia normonatraemia should be achieved in less than 24 hours.
   D Hypertensive encephalopathy is associated with a diastolic blood pressure of 130 mmHg or greater.

9.
   A Communicating hydrocephalus can result in herniation.
   B The absence of papilloedema is a reliable sign that intracranial pressure is not elevated.

C Sixth nerve palsies are early signs of herniation.

D Mannitol is used in the management of herniation.

10. Brain death

A Cortical integrity is assessed as part of the UK brain death protocol.

B A brain stem is a prerequisite to life.

C One examination of the brain-stem reflexes is sufficient to diagnose brain death.

D Apnoea is a prerequisite for the diagnosis of brain death.

12. Disorders that affect the spinal cord

Objectives

This chapter is concerned with pathologies that affect the spinal cord. The areas covered are:

- The presentation of spinal cord disease
- Transverse myelitis
- Anterior spinal artery thrombosis
- Intrinsic cord lesions
- Extrinsic cord lesions
- Traumatic cord damage
- Management of chronic myelopathy

The spinal cord is an important source of much disability. Most of the disability in patients with MS is due to their spinal cord lesions. Failure to diagnose and treat appropriately spinal cord disorders is one of the major pitfalls to the budding neurologist. The management of acute cord compression is discussed in Chapter 20.

Presentation

The final stages of spinal cord disease are dramatic, ending in either paraplegia or quadriplegia, but the initial presentation may be subtle and it is at this stage that intervention may be most beneficial. The hallmarks of spinal cord disease are bilateral weakness, a sensory level and autonomic failure (Table 12.1).

The presentation of intrinsic and extrinsic pathologies usually differs. With *lesions intrinsic to the cord*, such as demyelination, the first symptoms may be subtle changes in autonomic function, such as urgency of micturition, a tendency to constipation or a difficulty in maintaining erections. This may be followed by paraesthesiae which is often in the tips of the fingers and toes mimicking a peripheral neuropathy. Unlike the latter Lhermitte's sign may be present. Actually the sign is a symptom in that when the patient flexes their neck, traction on the cord may induce a sensation like electricity running down their back and there may be a transient worsening of their paraesthesiae. The sensory complaints are often followed by motor complaints, such as weakness and stiffness in the legs. The legs may be noticed to jump spontaneously, particularly at night, though this has to be differentiated from the normal phenomenon of an occasional myoclonic jerk in drowsiness.

Extrinsic pathologies usually announce themselves with pain. The pain is at the level of the pathology and may radiate round the trunk as

---

Bilateral weakness
Sensory level
Autonomic
   Bowel
   Bladder
   Sexual dysfunction

Table 12.1 Cardinal features of cord disease

the lesion irritates a nerve root (radiculopathy). The nature of the lesion, its rapidity of growth and location will determine the course of events, but symptoms are often predominantly motor. If the process is gradual there may be a gradual increasing of tone in the legs with stiffness and later weakness developing. More rapidly progressive lesions in the cervical cord may start with monoplegia in one arm, followed by the leg on the same side, then the other leg and finally all four limbs. This is why it is worth considering cord disease in a patient with hemiplegia when there is no facial involvement and no evidence of pathology above the foramen magnum. Sensory loss usually follows the motor deficit in extrinsic lesions with the development of a sensory level. The apparent sensory level is often lower than the pathological process. Not infrequently this results in doctors imaging the thoracic spine, but failing to look at the cervical spine where the problem lies. The other trap in assessing sensory levels is that the dermatomal level for the localization of the lesion is not where a pin prick can be perceived, but where the sensation returns to normal. Finally, in compressive lesions, bladder, bowel and sexual function will be compromised. These functions have to be specifically asked about and in some detail, despite the doctor's embarrassment. Once a patient is quadriplegic and doubly incontinent for 24 hours the chances of getting any useful recovery is very low.

Spinal shock

Initially after damage to the spinal cord there is flaccidity and hyporeflexia. It takes time (hours to weeks) for the circuits that underlie hyperreflexia and increased tone to be established in the spinal cord. I missed a case of cord compression because of this phenomenon. It is a salutary lesson preferably learnt from a book.

Brown–Séquard syndrome

This describes the findings in hemisection of the cord. Not infrequently, elements of the Brown–Séquard syndrome are found in

Ipsilateral weakness
Ipsilateral posterior column loss
Vibration
Joint position sense
Contralateral spinothalamic loss
Pin prick
Temperature

Table 12.2 The Brown–Séquard syndrome

patients with cord pathology predominantly on one side. The main characteristics of the syndrome are weakness and pyramidal signs below the lesion on the same side, loss of posterior column sensory modalities (vibration and joint position sense) below the lesion on the same side and loss of spinothalamic sensation (pain and temperature) on the other side below the lesion (Table 12.2). One might find a patient with back pain, a weak leg and reduced pin prick sensation in the other leg. To the uninitiated this constellation might cause great confusion, but once the thought 'Brown–Séquard' passes through your mind the clouds of uncertainty should lift.

Transverse myelitis

Myelitis means inflammation of the cord; transverse means across it. Transverse myelitis is demyelination across the cord, which is often preceded by a viral infection. In about half of the cases it will be the harbinger of multiple sclerosis. It usually comes on over a few days and can result in the full gamut of signs and symptoms seen in cord transection. Despite its severity there is usually recovery, often rapid and complete. Patients frequently require urinary catheterization for retention during the acute phase. As well as general nursing care physiotherapy should be initiated early. Particular care should be directed to maintaining full range of movement. The Achilles tendons will rapidly shorten if the feet are left in dorsiflexion. High dose methyl prednisolone often shortens the period of disability (500 mg a day for 5 days), but probably does not have much effect on long-term prognosis.

As well as MS and postviral transverse myelitis it is worth considering rarer causes of myelitis such as mycoplasma, tuberculosis and lysteria as such infections will require specific treatment. The cord will have to be imaged (MRI or complete myelogram) to exclude structural lesions and the spinal fluid needs examining. In demyelination transverse myelitis the CSF should either be normal or have up to 20 lymphocytes in it. Occasionally hundreds of lymphocytes and a few polymorphs are present, but this should prompt a search for more esoteric and potentially treatable infectious causes.

Acute necrotizing myelitis

This may be the aggressive end of the spectrum of transverse myelitis, but the patient is systemically unwell, often with a fever. There is back pain and the CSF is reactive with polymorphs and an elevated protein. It is difficult initially to differentiate it from an abscess or TB, but early high dose steroid treatment may be important in influencing recovery.

Vacuolar myelopathy

HIV infection is associated with a vacuolar myelopathy. This usually presents fairly late in the course of the disease and seems to be a direct consequence of the HIV virus itself. It often occurs in the presence of the AIDS dementia. There are pyramidal signs in the lower extremities with loss of continence. The sensory level is often indistinct on the trunk. It is progressive and has not been proven to respond to any treatment.

Anterior spinal artery thrombosis

The spinal cord is supplied by an anterior spinal artery and two posterior spinal arteries. The anterior spinal artery supplies the anterior two-thirds of the spinal cord. It is formed by branches of the vertebral arteries and re-

supplied down its length by intercostal arteries. In the lower part at a variable level is found the great anterior radicular artery of Adamkiewicz. In a hypotensive episode the upper thoracic cord is particularly vulnerable and may infarct. In addition, the anterior spinal artery may be subject to atheroma or emboli and its supplying arteries may be involved in similar processes or dissection of the aorta. This results in the anterior spinal artery syndrome with the anterior two-thirds of the cord being infarcted. Patients often complain of sudden onset of severe back pain followed by loss of strength in the legs. They are usually in retention of urine. The most characteristic feature of the syndrome is the pattern of sensory loss. Spinothalamic modalities (pain and temperature) are lost, but posterior column modalities (vibration and joint position sense) are retained to a variable degree. Initially there is spinal shock with flaccidity and reduced reflexes. The prognosis is often poor.

Intrinsic cord lesions

The commonest intrinsic cord lesion is demyelination as in transverse myelitis. Additional intrinsic cord pathologies are syrinx, astrocytoma, ependymoma, subacute combined degeneration of the cord (B_{12} deficiency) and arteriovenous malformations (Table 12.3).

Syrinx

Syrinx is a curious condition in which the central portion of the cord cavitates. In the cord this process is called syringomyelia, when it extends rostrally into the medulla it is called syringobulbia. Syrinx may be secondary to

Demyelination
Syrinx
Ependymoma
Astrocytoma
SACDC (B_{12} deficiency)
Arteriovenous malformation

Table 12.3 Intrinsic cord pathologies

Case history

Claire Bucknall was a 19-year-old student of psychology who was admitted as an emergency, having developed weakness of the legs over a 24-hour period, to the point she could not stand. In addition, she had lost sensation up to her umbilicus and was having difficulty passing urine. Three weeks previously she had had a bad cold. On examination she had a flaccid paraplegia with loss of joint position sense, vibration and reduced pain sensation in the legs. Pin prick sensation returned to normal just above the umbilicus. She had a palpable bladder. The deep tendon reflexes were reduced in her legs and the plantar responses were silent.

An MR of the spine was unremarkable. Examination of the spinal fluid demonstrated 15 lymphocytes. She was give a 5-day course of 500 mg methylprednisolone intravenously. Within 2 days there was improvement in her condition and by the end of the week she was walking normally. Oligoclonal bands came back as negative and an MRI of the brain was normal. At follow up 6 months later she was symptomatically normal. A diagnosis of a postviral transverse myelitis was made.

trauma, intrinsic tumours, arachnoiditis, or in association with a Chiari malformation, but often it is idiopathic. Various theories as to the cause abound, such that it is due to pressure waves travelling down the central canal of the cord, but I feel they fall squarely within neuromythology. Patients present with gradual onset of sensory loss, predominantly spinothalamic modalities, and lower motor neurone signs in the segments at the level of the syrinx. Below the syrinx are upper motor neurone signs. In addition, sphincter and sensory disturbances below the syrinx occur. The classical description is of wasting in the hands with a cape-like sensory loss to pin prick over the shoulders. Patients may have burns on their hands from loss of pain and temperature sensation. The condition is usually slowly progressive. Various surgical procedures can be tried, such as shunting the syrinx, decompressing the level of the syrinx or blocking the

central canal above the syrinx; all have variable results.

Ependymoma

Ependymomas have already been mentioned in Chapter 11. The central canal of the cord is lined with ependymal cells which can develop malignant change. Sixty per cent of intrinsic spinal cord tumours are of this histological type. These tumours then act as an intrinsic mass in the cord, causing all the symptoms we have previously discussed. The diagnosis of an intrinsic cord tumour will be made on MRI (or myelography), but the histological diagnosis is a little more problematic as biopsy will often worsen the clinical situation. Treatment is with steroids and radiotherapy. The prognosis is not good.

Astrocytoma

These are the next commonest intrinsic cord tumours. They may be very slowly progressive and are often associated with a syrinx. Their treatment is problematic as they are so slowly growing, but often involves radiotherapy.

Subacute combined degeneration of the cord (SACDC) (B$_{12}$ deficiency)

This is a rare complication of B$_{12}$ deficiency. There is a gradual development of a cord syndrome with spasticity in the legs with extensor plantar responses and often absent ankle jerks. There is frequently profound loss of posterior column modalities (vibration and joint position sense). The majority of the pathology is in the cord, but there is debate about the coexistence of a peripheral neuropathy. This would be the simplest explanation of the loss of reflexes at the ankles. SACDC is usually a complication of pernicious anaemia, but can occur in nutritional B$_{12}$ deficiency in vegans. It is treated with B$_{12}$ injections, but the response is variable.

Arteriovenous malformation (AVM)

It is not clear if AVMs should be classified as extrinsic or intrinsic as the majority of them lie on the surface of the cord. They consist of a short cut between the arterial and venous blood systems without a capillary bed between. This results in a high blood flow through these abnormalities and they tend to grow. They consist of hypertrophied and tortuous vessels. Symptoms are due to compression and more importantly ischaemia. The exact mechanism is not clear, but a steal phenomenon might be important (blood is stolen from the normal circuitry for this low resistance path). An additional factor may be venous hypertension resulting in poor flow in the capillary bed. While they can bleed their usual presentation is of a slowly progressive myelopathy, which often proceeds step wise and may have remissions and exacerbations. MRI of the cord is not particularly good at present in detecting these abnormalities. The only clue may be on conventional myelography, where serpeginous shadows from the vessels may be seen over the cord. The definitive test is spinal angiography, though this is hazardous as it may precipitate cord infarction and some idea of the level is required as cannulization of all the intercostal arteries is laborious and dangerous. Treatment is surgical or via embolization. Often it is not very satisfactory.

Extrinsic cord lesions

The extrinsic cord lesions cause cord compression. This may be slowly progressive and at times patients with few symptoms may be seen with only a wisp of cord left sneaking past near obliteration of the canal. If the pathology is rapidly progressive the clinical course can be rapid, at times changing from near normality to quadriplegia overnight. The more common cases of cord compression are given in Table 12.4.

Cervical spondylosis

Cervical degenerative disease is almost ubiquitous as the years advance. Whether the cord

Cervical spondylosis
Metastasis
Neurofibroma
Meningioma
Abscess
Haematoma

Table 12.4 Extrinsic causes of cord compression

becomes involved depends on the original diameter of the spinal canal, horizontal slippage of vertebrae on one another (subluxation), disc herniation and bony growth. Cervical degenerative disease usually presents with pain in the neck often radiating into the shoulders and arms. There may be lower motor neurone signs and sensory symptoms from impingement on the cervical roots. The myelopathy is usually slowly progressive, though there can be sudden exacerbations, particularly if the patient falls. Often there is a spastic paraparesis with hyper-reflexia and extensor plantar responses. Sensory and autonomic features are not prominent initially. Often a conservative approach is the best management, but surgery should be considered if there is disability developing, particularly in younger patients.

Metastasis

Metastases are the most common cause of non-traumatic acute cord compression. The most common are prostate, lung, breast, thyroid and myeloma. Spinal metastases are often the initial presentation of malignancy. The patients usually have back pain, frequently with a radicular component preceding the cord symptoms. Prognosis depends on the underlying neoplasm and the general condition of the patients, but most importantly from the neurological point of view the degree of disability at the time of initiation of therapy. There are delays between initial symptoms and treatment, the most significant delay usually being due to the patient's reticence about seeking medical advice. However, there is often some avoidable delay once the patient has presented to the medical profession. It i important that the diagnosis is considered and that once considered appropriate investigations are undertaken at speed. The time between presentation and treatment should ideally not be more than 24 hours. The most important investigation is imaging of the cord. Ideally this should be by MR, but where this is not available conventional myelography followed by CT of the area around the blockage provides excellent images. Once the abnormality has been detected histological confirmation of the cause is required. This is usually performed by CT-guided needle biopsy, but open biopsy at laminectomy is sometimes required. Treatment consists of steroids followed by either surgery or more commonly radiotherapy.

Neurofibroma and meningioma

Neurofibroma and meningioma are the most common benign tumours causing cord compression. Both usually occur extramedullary, but intradural, i.e. outside the cord, but inside the dural sac. Meningiomas are more common in the thoracic cord and also occur more often in women than men. Neurofibromas can occur singularly or as part of neurofibromatosis. They can occur anywhere along the cord and classically can form a dumbbell shape if they are poking through the intervertebral foramen with half the tumour within the spinal canal and half outside.

Rarer causes of cord compression

Rarer causes of cord compression are abscess, haematoma and thoracic disc herniation. Extradural abscess formation is often associated with an infected intervertebral disc. Patients particularly at risk are the elderly and intravenous drug users. Haematomas can arise spontaneously, but are often associated with abnormal clotting, either therapeutic or not.

Traumatic cord damage

It is beyond the scope of this book to describe the correct management of trauma victims, but it is worth emphasizing that head and neck injuries often coexist. Patients should not be moved until the neck has been stabilized. Patients with neck pain who have sustained a head injury, particularly if they have had neurological symptoms in the limbs, should be presumed to have a cervical spine fracture until proven otherwise. I have seen two patients walk into casualty about a week after a head injury complaining of neck pain who proved to have unstable fractures, which had been held in place by spasm of the neck muscles.

Management of chronic myelopathy

A large proportion of the disability seen in neurological practice is due to cord damage and the management of chronic myelopathy is an important aspect of neurological care. As mentioned above, cord damage results in weakness, spasticity, loss of sensation and loss of autonomic control.

Currently there is little one can do for the weakness directly apart from allowing the patient to make maximum use of the power still available. Physiotherapists and occupational therapists are skilled in maximizing this potential and the appropriate referrals should be made. Mechanical aids such as splints for foot drop may be of some help and will usually be suggested by the physiotherapist. The appropriateness of additional ambulatory aids that use the strength in the arms, such as walking sticks, elbow crutches, zimmer frames or a wheel chair will be assessed. Physiotherapy has a major role in the prevention of contractures (shortening of tendons).

Physiotherapy can have an impact on spasticity in the legs, but medical therapy also has a role. There has to be a balance struck between reduction in spasticity and increased weakness. Some patients are dependent on the stiffness in their legs to be able to walk. There are three drugs which are clinically useful in the treatment of spasms and spasticity and these are baclofen, diazepam and dantrolene. Baclofen (a GABA agonist) is the most useful; a small dose should be used initially, gradually building up until maximum benefit or unacceptable side effects, such as drowsiness, are reached.

While nothing can currently be done about loss of sensation some patients are troubled by abnormal sensations (dysaesthesiae). These can sometimes be modified with amitriptyline or carbamazepine.

Bladder care is important in chronic spinal cord pathology. There is always the danger of sepsis from urinary tract infections and this is a cause of significant morbidity and mortality. Where control of bladder function is lost intermittent self-catheterization is probably one of the best solutions where the patient or a carer has the capacity to perform this. Another alternative is a permanent indwelling catheter. Bowel function can be managed by the use of aperients and enemas.

MCQs for Chapter 12

The MCQs are either true T or false F. The answers are given in Appendix 3. Negatively mark your answers; a point for a correct answer, deduct a point for an incorrect response. If you score 24 or more you pass.

1. **Cardinal features of cord disease are:**
   A Dysarthria.
   B A sensory level.
   C Sexual dysfunction.
   D Diplopia.

2. **In the Brown–Séquard syndrome:**
   A Lower motor neurone signs are found in the legs.
   B Vibration loss is contralateral to the lesion.
   C Weakness is ipsilateral to the lesion.
   D Pin prick sensation is predominantly reduced contralateral to the lesion.

3. **The blood supply to the cord:**
   A Is mostly via the posterior spinal artery.
   B The cervical cord is supplied by the artery of Adamkiewicz.
   C Vibration sensation is often preserved in anterior spinal artery thrombosis.
   D Reflexes may be initially reduced in spinal infarction.

4.
   A Subacute combined degeneration of the cord is due to a thiamine deficiency.
   B The most common intrinsic cord tumours are astrocytomas.
   C The prognosis with a spinal cord ependymoma is good.
   D Absent ankle jerks can be a feature of B_{12} deficiency.

5.
   A Cervical degenerative disease is usually associated with pain.
   B Spinal meningiomas are commonly found in the thoracic spine.

   C Intravenous drug users are at risk of extradural abscesses.
   D Neurofibromas are tumours of the arachnoid.

6. **Traumatic cord damage:**
   A May occur on moving the patient.
   B Is commonly associated with head injury.
   C Can be excluded with plane cervical films.
   D Is usually associated with pain.

7. **Spinal metastasis:**
   A Is the most common cause of non-traumatic cord compression.
   B Back pain is a late feature.
   C MR is the optimal method of imaging the cord.
   D The commonest definitive treatment is decompressive laminectomy.

8. **Transverse myelitis:**
   A May be the first harbinger of multiple sclerosis.
   B Urinary symptoms are unusual.
   C Good recovery is rare.
   D A few additional lymphocytes are often seen in the CSF.

9. **Syrinx:**
   A May be associated with trauma.
   B Lower motor neurone signs are common in the feet.
   C Spinothalamic loss is typical at the level of the syrinx.
   D May be associated with a Chiari malformation.

10. **Arteriovenous malformations in the cord:**
    A Arteriovenous malformations usually resolve spontaneously.
    B They usually present with a step-wise progressive myelopathy.
    C The definitive investigation is spinal angiography.
    D Embolization is sometimes undertaken.

13. Disorders of roots and nerves

Objectives

This chapter covers the peripheral nervous system. Particular areas covered include:

- Radiculopathies
- Plexopathies
- Mononeuritis multiplex
- Mononeuritis
- Distal sensory motor neuropathies
- Pure motor neuropathies
- Spinal muscular atrophies

In 1908 Rivers and Head reported the results of a human experiment (A human experiment in nerve division, *Brain* 1908; **31**: 323–50). Henry Head had allowed his radial nerve to be cut in order to observe the sensory deficits and the return of sensation. This was an extraordinarily brave act in the pre-penicillin era and demonstrates beyond all reasonable doubt that the peripheral nervous system is of interest and intellectual challenge to some of the greatest neurological minds. That I do not find myself in their company is of some personal regret, but I do appreciate that a working knowledge of the peripheral nervous system is of great utilitarian importance to the practising neurologist as a high proportion of patients have problems in this area.

Radiculopathies

The peripheral nervous system is attached to the cord by two rami, ventral (carrying motor fibres) and dorsal (carrying sensory fibres). These rami join together to form the nerve root within the spinal canal. The nerve root then exits through the intervertebral foramen and either forms a segmental nerve with dorsal and ventral branches or joins in the cervical or lumbosacral nerve plexuses. Root damage or irritation (radiculopathy) is one of the most common neurological complaints (Table 13.1).

Herniated nucleus pulposus (HNP)

This may be the best of all possible worlds, but human beings have a number of design faults, the appendix, the female reproductive system, and the spinal column. This flexible long-

Herniated nucleus pulposus
Malignancy
Carcinomatous/lymphomatous meningitis
Bony metastasis
Infection
Direct viral
Meningitis
Epidural abscess
Arachnoiditis, e.g. Myodil
Bone disease
Osteoporosis
Paget's disease
Trauma

Table 13.1 Causes of radiculopathy

itudinal structure is perfectly adequate if you are a cow on all four limbs, but once you spend most of your life upright it has to perform in compression. It is composed of vertebral bodies, which are like building blocks, between which are intervertebral discs, which act as shock absorbers. Facet joints and ligaments hold the column together. The intervertebral discs consist of a fibrous outer ring with a squishy centre. As these discs are subjected to repeated compression and begin to degenerate the squishy centre can ooze out. This is called a herniated nucleus pulposus or slipped disc in the vernacular. The direction in which the nucleus herniates determines how much trouble it causes, but not infrequently it herniates laterally into the intervertebral canal squashing the emerging root. This causes pain, which is usually in the low back (the commonest site for a HNP) and radiates along the course of the nerve root. Patients call this sciatica, but the pathology is not in the sciatic nerve, but one of the roots that make it up. This can be demonstrated by doing a straight leg raise. If the leg is passively raised with the patient lying on their back at some point the patient experiences discomfort. In normal individuals this is at about 90° and the pain is felt in the back of the knee. In a patient with a radiculopathy it may be at 30°, is excruciating and is felt in the lower back. Fortunately most HNPs resolve spontaneously. Patients may require analgesics, bed rest on a firm bed or the floor and should be careful about lifting in the future. If the pain is unremitting for over 6 weeks or there are neurological signs then a discectomy is worth considering.

Malignancy

Malignancy not infrequently announces itself with radicular pain, but most radicular pain is secondary to degenerative disease. This is because degenerative disease is almost ubiquitous while malignancy is a life event in only about half the population and causes back pain only rarely. There are three sites where malignancy gives rise to radicular symptoms. The first is within the spinal canal. Carcinomatous or lymphomatous meningitis has already been mentioned in Chapter 11. The sheets of malignant cells can pick off roots or cranial nerves. Second, metastases can occur in the vertebral bodies. As the vertebral body is destroyed the intervertebral foramen is often involved, either directly by tumour, or indirectly by collapsing bony architecture. Third, paraspinal masses may involve roots on their way to the plexi. Root involvement with cancer will usually present with pain in the sensory distribution of the root. As the malignancy progresses sensory and motor loss will become demonstrable. After a diagnosis has been made radiotherapy is the usual palliative therapy. Steroids can also be useful.

Infection

Viruses can directly infect nerve roots. The most common is herpes simplex (cold sores). Recurrent vesicular eruptions around the mouth are due to type 1, while genital herpes is either due to type 1 or 2. The initial response to exposure may be severe with generalized symptoms as well as acute pain and inflammation in the area affected. During recurrent attacks the symptoms are less severe. Virus is shed from the vesicles, but may be present at other times. Transmission is by direct contact and exposure to HSV1 is almost 100% by the time of adulthood. Acyclovir cream can reduce symptoms in recurrent attacks; systemic treatment with acyclovir may be needed for severe initial attacks or in immunocompromised individuals. The first indication of a further attack is usually paraesthesiae in the distribution of a nerve. Herpes zoster is another common virus. After an initial attack with chicken pox the virus hides from immunological attack in the nerve roots. A variable time later, often at times of general debilitation, the virus becomes active again and effects a root distribution. The first symptoms are paraesthesiae followed by pain, which can be excruciating. A few days to a week later vesicles appear in the dermatomal area of the affected root ('shingles'). Over the next few weeks the vesicles heal, often leaving brown papular scars. The pain usually resolves, but can remain as a post-herpetic neuralgia. Acyclovir can be of some assistance in treating the initial attack and should be given systemically in immunocompromised individuals to stop viraemic spread. The postherpetic neuralgia is difficult to treat. Carbamazepine, amitriptyline and capsaicin cream are the usual mainstays of medical treatment.

In patients with AIDS a lumbosacral radiculopathy secondary to cytomegalovirus is increasingly being recognized. This is treated with ganciclovir, though with mixed results.

Bacterial infections can cause radiculopathies in two main ways. First, infection of the disc space can lead to epidural abscess infection and this can impinge on the root at the intervertebral foramen. Second, within the subarachnoid space roots are vulnerable to meningitis. This is unusual in bacterial meningitis, where cranial nerve damage is much more common, but the 'funnies' such as TB and mycoplasma can cause radiculopathies.

Other causes

Bone disease, other than degenerative conditions, can involve the roots. Paget's disease can give a sacral plexopathy if the sacrum is involved and roots travelling through it are compressed. Osteoporosis not infrequently leads to vertebral collapse. This may be asymptomatic, but often results in severe pain, some of which is radicular in origin. The pain settles spontaneously after a few weeks. Trauma can result in evulsion of nerve roots, particularly traction injuries to the upper limb. If the roots have been completely evulsed there will be no recovery.

Plexopathies

In the cervical and lumbosacral regions the roots form a nerve plexus. Out of these plexi run the nerves that supply the limbs. As a variety of roots contribute to each nerve there is a considerable degree of complexity within each of these plexi. As an alternative to memorizing the London Underground there may be some merit in learning these natural spaghetti junctions, but for practical purposes I find it more secure to look them up in *Aids to the Examination of the Peripheral Nervous System* (Baillière Tindall, Editorial Committee of The Guarantors of Brain 1986, London) whenever I wish to localize a lesion in a plexus.

Brachial neuralgia

This is also known as brachial amyotrophy, neuralgic amyotrophy, Parsonage Turner syndrome and idiopathic brachial plexus neuropathy. It starts with severe pain in the shoulder which comes on over a few hours. The pain then subsides over about 3 to 6 weeks. After a few days weakness develops in the arm. In addition there is often some sensory disturbance, though this is a less prominent feature. As the weeks go by there is wasting in the muscles affected. Most patients make a near full recovery, though this may take a couple of years. Like most ideopathic conditions it has been attributed to a preceding viral infection. Management is with analgesics, carbamazepine and amitriptyline for the pain and physiotherapy to maintain range of movement and prevent the development of a frozen shoulder. As a point of neurotrivia there is a rare recurrent and familial form in which there is 'tomaculous' (sausage-shaped) change to the myelin sheaths on teased sural nerve biopsies. The same change can be seen in patients with familial recurrent pressure palsies.

Pancoast's plexopathy

Pancoast's tumour is usually a squamous cell carcinoma of the apex of the lung. This tumour can spread to involve the lower cervical roots or the lower parts of the brachial plexus. In addition, the stellate ganglion may be involved, causing Horner's syndrome. It presents with severe, unremitting pain radiating down the arm with neurological signs referable to the lower parts of the plexus. Palliative treatment with radiotherapy is the only effective form of therapy.

Cervical rib

The seventh cervical vertebrae may have an elongated transverse process that forms a cervical rib, or there may be only a fibrous band in place of the rib. Either of these congenital abnormalities can compress the lower cords of the brachial plexus causing a sensory disturbance on the ulnar border of the hand and wasting of the thenar eminence. There may in addition be vascular involvement. In the past it has been difficult to diagnose, but MRI of the plexus will demonstrate distortion and surgery in such patients has good results.

Diabetic amyotrophy

The exact cause of this syndrome is not well understood, but in some mature onset diabetics there can be a relatively sudden onset of severe pain in a lower limb associated with proximal weakness and wasting. This has been attributed to a vascular event in the lumbar plexus. The pain resolves, but although there may be some recovery of power it is usually incomplete. Although onset is usually unilateral, many patients ultimately have bilateral involvement.

Mononeuritis multiplex

This is an oxymoron, for how can something that is mono be multi, but it well describes a recognized clinical syndrome. The clinical picture is of a patient who has individual peripheral neuropathies, usually scattered throughout the body and time. For example, a radial neuropathy on the right can be followed by a common peroneal neuropathy on the left and median neuropathy on the left. Diabetes is by far the most common cause of mononeuritis multiplex, but a predominantly sensory distal polyneuropathy is the most common diabetic neuropathy. Some of the causes of mononeuritis multiplex are given in Table 13.2.

Diabetes mellitus
Vasculitis
   Systemic lupus erythematosus
   Rheumatoid
   Polyarteritis nodosa
   Weigner's granulomatosus
Hereditary pressure sensitive neuropathy
Sarcoid
Leprosy

Table 13.2 Causes of mononeuritis multiplex

Mononeuritis

All the causes of mononeuritis multiplex can cause a mononeuritis. Additional causes of mononeuritis are trauma of various sorts and pressure palsies. There are various points on the body where peripheral nerves are particularly likely to be exposed to pressure damage. The most common is the carpal tunnel, but the ulnar nerve can be compressed at the elbow, the radial as it runs round the humerus and the common peroneal as it runs over the head of the fibula (see Chapter 9).

Carpal tunnel syndrome

The median nerve runs through the carpal tunnel as it gains access to the hand. Compression of the nerve in the tunnel gives rise to the syndrome, which is usually idiopathic, but has a number of medical associations (Table 13.3). Patients complain of paraesthesiae in the hand which is characteristically worse at night. There may be frank pain which can radiate proximally as far as the shoulder. In addition there is a weakening of grip in the hand with patients complaining of dropping things, or not being able to unscrew jars. On examination there may be wasting of the outer thenar

Idiopathic
Pregnancy
Myxoedema
Rheumatoid arthritis
Acromegaly

Table 13.3 Causes of carpal tunnel syndrome

eminence and sensory loss confined to the median nerve distribution, often with splitting of the fourth finger. Opposition of the thumb and little finger may be weak. Percussion over the carpal tunnel may produce paraesthesia in the median distribution (Tinel's sign). If the wrists are forcibly hyperextended the symptoms can often be reproduced (Phalen's sign). The diagnosis should be confirmed electrophysiologically. Splints can give temporary relief, but most established cases require surgical division of the transverse carpal ligament.

Distal sensory motor neuropathies

Most neuropathies are of this type. They start distally with both sensory and motor component, but the sensory is often more prominent and presents a 'glove and stocking' sensory loss. The deep tendon reflexes are reduced or lost, particularly in demyelinating neuropathies with a sensory component. These neuropathies can be differentiated into axonal and demyelinating depending on the pathological process. This differentiation can usually be made by electrophysiological examination (see Chapter 10).

Axonal peripheral neuropathies

All the causes of mononeuritis multiplex (Table 13.2) can cause a distal axonal neuropathy if a sufficient number of peripheral nerves are involved. In addition, amyloidosis, Lyme disease and the majority of toxins (usually drugs, Table 13.4) that act on nerves cause axonal damage. Motor neurone disease can cause an axonal motor neuropathy, but is almost invariably associated with upper motor neurone signs (see p. 155).

Demyelinating peripheral neuropathies

The most common causes of demyelinating peripheral neuropathies are given in Table 13.5. The only demyelinating peripheral

Ethanol
Cisplatin
Vincristine
Phenytoin
Colchicine
Isoniazid
Dapsone
Ethambutol
Amioderone (demyelinating)
Gold
Metronidazole

Table 13.4 Drugs that can cause a neuropathy

Guillain–Barré syndrome
Chronic inflammatory demyelinating polyneuropathy
Paraproteinaemic neuropathy
Hereditary motor and sensory neuropathy
Inherited metabolic diseases
Multifocal motor neuropathy with conduction block
Amioderone neuropathy

Table 13.5 Demyelinating peripheral neuropathies

neuropathy commonly encountered is the Guillain –Barré Syndrome.

Guillain–Barré syndrome (GBS)
Guillain–Barré syndrome is an acute demyelinating polyneuropathy and is often postinfection. There is often a history of an upper respiratory tract infection or gastrointestinal disturbance between 10 days and 3 weeks prior to the onset of symptoms. The initial symptoms are usually tingling in the extremities and these abnormal sensations move proximally as the disease progresses. The next symptom is often weakness in the legs which patients may describe as wobbliness or feeling as if their legs have gone to jelly. The condition can progress from being asymptomatic to quadriplegia requiring respiratory support within a couple of days.

The most important differentiation is between GBS and cord pathology, and this can be difficult. Initially the reflexes may be preserved in GBS and reduced or lost in spinal shock. There should be a sensory level in a myelopathy, but the shield of preserved sensation on the chest of a patient with GBS may mimic this. If there is doubt the cord will have to be imaged.

In GBS the CSF protein should be elevated, though this can take a couple of days. Usually there are only a normal number of lymphocytes present in the CSF. Lymphocyte counts in the teens should alert the clinician to the possibility of concurrent HIV infection and counts above this should cause reconsideration of the diagnosis. Initially electrophysiology in GBS may be remarkably normal, but later conduction block and slowing are demonstrable. If there has been a significant amount of axonal damage denervation will be demonstrable on EMG and this indicates a poorer prognosis. Management is initially directed at supporting the patient. Respiratory embarrassment used to be a major cause of mortality, but this should not be the case now. A vital capacity of one litre or less should prompt movement to an ITU (see Chapter 20). Patients may well have difficulties swallowing and should be fed nasogastrically should that occur. Specific therapy consists of either pooled human immunoglobulin or plasma exchange. Most patients will have plateaued by 2 weeks and if they continue to deteriorate after a month then the diagnosis is in doubt.

Progressive demyelinating polyneuropathy of more than 6 weeks duration raises the possibility of it being *chronic inflammatory demyelinating polyneuropathy*. Unlike GBS this responds to steroids. Most patients with GBS make a good recovery, though this may be slow. The mortality is surprisingly high at about 15%. While some of this may be due to suboptimal management the complications of intensive care (pneumonia, line sepsis, pulmonary embolism) take their toll. In addition, in bad GBS there is autonomic involvement. This is particularly difficult to manage as there can be wild fluctuations in blood pressure and heart rate. Medical treatment with beta-blockers is often tried. I would advise early insertion of a pacing wire if bradyarrhythmias are present, the use of position for the control of blood pressure and extreme caution in stimulating the pharynx during sucking out as this can precipitate a parasympathetic mediated cardiac arrest.

Case history

Mrs Hanley was a 65-year-old retired cleaner who was transferred from St Elsewhere's district general hospital having been admitted 1 week previously. She was admitted to St Elsewhere's having gone off her legs over 4 days. In addition she had had diarrhoea 10 days prior to developing her neurological condition. Over the week at St Elsewhere's she had deteriorated with progressive weakness in all four limbs and difficulty swallowing. She complained of sensory disturbance in her limbs, but there was little demonstrable sensory loss. A psychiatric diagnosis had been entertained, but her worsening respiratory status had prompted her transfer.

On examination she had a flaccid quadriplegia, bilateral facial weakness and a glove and stocking sensory loss to pin prick. No deep tendon reflexes were elicitable. Her vital capacity was 0.5 l. She was transferred to ITU and fed nasogastrically. Her CSF protein was elevated at 2 g/l and electrophysiology confirmed Guillian–Barré syndrome. She was given a 5-day course of intravenous immunoglobulin. By the end of the week she was beginning to improve. She did not require mechanical ventilation. Her recovery was complicated by a chest infection and hyponatraemia. After 6 weeks she was sitting out and able to weight bear on her legs. She was transferred back to St Elsewhere's to continue her rehabilitation. At follow up at 6 months she was living independently at home, but still had some distal weakness in the legs and was troubled by dysaesthesiae.

Pure motor neuropathies

Pure motor neuropathies can provide a diagnostic challenge. Their differential diagnosis is given in Table 13.6. In recent years it has been recognized that some patients with pure lower motor neurone signs, who formerly might have been diagnosed as having motor neurone disease (see Chapter 19) have a multifocal motor neuropathy with conduction block. The appropriate electrophysiological examination will make this differentiation. These

Motor neurone disease
Multifocal motor neuropathy with conduction block
Guillain–Barré syndrome
Porphyria
Poisoning
Lead
Dapsone
Organophosphates

Table 13.6 Causes of motor peripheral neuropathies

patients get worse on steroids, but at least some improve on cyclophosphamide or intravenous pooled human immunoglobulin.

Spinal muscular atrophies

These are a rare group of genetic disorders characterized by degeneration of motor neurones in the spinal cord and brain stem. They produce a chronic denervating picture on EMG. Their classification is controversial, but at present is based on age of onset, rate of progression and muscle groups affected. In children there is a rapidly progressive autosomal recessive form with death within 3 years called Werdnig–Hoffmann disease (incidence 1/25 000 births) and a chronic form called Kugelberg–Welander disease. A satisfactory classification of these disorders will have to await the identification of the responsible genes.

MCQs for Chapter 13

The MCQs are either true T or false F. The answers are given in Appendix 3. Negatively mark your answers; a point for a correct answer, deduct a point for an incorrect response. If you score 24 or more you pass.

1. **Causes of radiculopathies include:**
   A Vincristine.
   B Arachnoiditis.
   C Herniated nucleus pulposus.
   D Myxoedema.

2. **Infections and roots:**
   A Cold sores are due to herpes simplex virus type 2.
   B The first sign of shingles is a vesicular rash.
   C Cytomegalovirus can cause a lumbosacral radiculopathy in AIDS patients.
   D Meningitis can lead to radiculopathy.

3. **Plexopathies:**
   A Brachial neuralgia presents with pain.
   B Pancoast's tumour can cause Horner's syndrome.
   C Cervical ribs often cause sensory loss on the radial border of the hand.
   D The weakness in diabetic amyotrophy is predominantly distal.

4. **The causes of mononeuritis multiplex include:**
   A Polyarteritis nodosa.
   B Thyrotoxicosis.
   C Diabetes mellitus.
   D Trauma.

5. **Carpal tunnel syndrome:**
   A Involves the ulnar nerve.
   B Tinel's sign may be positive.

C Can be caused by myxoedema.
   D Can be caused by Weigner's granulomatosis.

6. **Neuropathies:**
   A Glove and stocking sensory loss is typical of radiculopathy.
   B Demyelination causes slowing of conduction.
   C Drugs usually cause demyelinating neuropathies.
   D Deep tendon reflexes are lost or reduced in neuropathies.

7. **Drugs that cause neuropathies include:**
   A Ethanol.
   B Penicillin.
   C Phenytoin.
   D Carbamazepine.

8. **Guillain–Barré syndrome:**
   A Is often preceded by a viral infection.
   B Has a mortality of less than 5%.
   C The initial differential diagnosis is with myelopathy.
   D Steroids are the treatment of choice.

9. **Pure motor neuropathies include:**
   A Multifocal motor neuropathy with conduction block.
   B Diabetes.
   C B_{12} deficiency.
   D Porphyria.

10. **Radiculopathies:**
    A Limited straight leg raise suggests a lumbosacral radiculopathy.
    B Surgery is usually the appropriate treatment for malignant radiculopathy.
    C The most common site for a herniated nucleus pulposus is the lower back.
    D Most herniated nuclei pulposi require surgery.

14. Disorders of the neuromuscular junction and muscle

Objectives

In this chapter we discuss the more important disorders of the neuromuscular junction and muscle. Particular areas covered include:

- Myasthenia gravis
- Lambert–Eaton myasthenic syndrome
- Botulism
- Neuromuscular blocking agents
- Muscular disease   Muscular dystrophies
                      Inflammatory myositises
                      Myopathies

As we continue our journey outwards from the cerebral cortex to the utter darkness and wailing and gnashing of the intellect we come across the neuromuscular junction (NMJ) and finally muscle. The physiology of the neuromuscular junction has been discussed in Chapter 10.

Disorders of the NMJ are limited in number and are relatively simple to understand (Table 14.1).

Myasthenia gravis (MG)

This is an autoimmune disorder where antibodies are directed against the α-subunit of

Myasthenia gravis
Lambert–Eaton myasthenic syndrome
Congenital myasthenia
Botulism
Neuromuscular blocking agents

Table 14.1 Disorders of the neuromuscular junction

the acetylcholine receptor that lies in the postsynaptic membrane. The antibodies cause a reduction in the number of functioning receptors. It has an incidence of about 5–10/100 000. Clinically patients present with weakness and fatiguability in their muscles. The weakness tends to fluctuate, being worse when the patient is tired. Diplopia is a common initial symptom, classically first noticed driving at night when the headlights of an oncoming car separate into two images. Other symptoms include ptosis, difficulty in lifting the arms, for example in combing the hair, dysphagia, and difficulty in climbing stairs. The mildest form is purely ocular MG with diplopia and ptosis. The most severe is generalized MG, where the limbs, swallowing and respiratory musculature may be involved. There are two broad categories of patients with MG, those in their twenties and thirties who are predominantly female and older patients in their sixties and seventies who are more likely to be male. The younger group are the classic autoimmune patients and may well have a family history of

Case history

Keith Etruria is a 35-year-old labourer in a lumber warehouse who presented with 2 months of diplopia, initially at night and 2 weeks of limb weakness. He had been unable to work for a week and was having difficulty walking any distance. On examination he had a fatiguable ptosis of his right eye and variable diplopia, particularly on upward gaze. There was proximal weakness in all four limbs that was fatiguable in the upper extremities. The deep tendon reflexes were all brisk and the sensory examination was normal. A clinical diagnosis of myasthenia gravis was made, confirmed by the electrophysiology and acetylcholine receptor antibody. Treatment with acetylcholine esterase inhibitors was only partially effective. He was started on 100 mg of prednisolone on alternate days and 2.5 mg/kg of azathioprine daily. After a week, just as his weakness began to deteriorate further he had a 5-day course of plasma exchange. Following this he began to improve. A CT scan of the thorax demonstrated a thymoma. He was discharged after 1 month with good power in the limbs, but not yet strong enough for his occupation. A thymectomy is planned for a couple of months' time when his myasthenia is well controlled.

other autoimmune problems such as thyroid disease, vitiligo or rheumatoid arthritis. The older patients often have an underlying thymoma which has induced the autoimmune process.

The examination of a patient with suspected MG will be directed to demonstrate fatiguability and weakness in affected muscles. While checking eye movements the position of maximum deviation should be maintained for a few seconds to see if diplopia can be induced. Ptosis should be specifically looked for. Particular attention should be paid to the relationship between the pupils and the upper lids. This should be the same on both sides. If the patient has bilateral ptosis this difference may not be apparent. If more than two-fifths of the pupil is covered by the upper lid, this is obviously dysfunctional and suggestive of

ptosis. The patient should be asked to look up for a few minutes to see if a fatiguable ptosis can be demonstrated. In the limbs it is often helpful to exercise one arm then compare the strength in the two sides, using the other as a control. The deep tendon reflexes in MG are normal or brisk, but after sustained contraction of a muscle they become reduced or absent. There should be no sensory changes in MG.

The most useful test for confirming the diagnosis is the acetylcholine receptor antibody titre. If positive the diagnosis is secure. In purely ocular myasthenia the antibody is negative in about half the cases. In generalized myasthenia about 30% will remain antibody negative. Electrophysiological testing can provide confirmatory evidence of a defect in neuromuscular transmission. There are two main tests, the repetitive stimulation or Jolly test and single fibre studies. The Jolly test involves recording the electrical response of muscle to a train of impulses sent down the motor nerve. In MG there is a decrement in response and this is the electrical equivalent to fatiguability. Single fibre EMG demonstrates blocking and jitter in disorders of neuromuscular transmission. Using a special needle the electrical activity of two fascicles of muscle from the same motor unit (see Chapter 10) can be recorded. In health, when one fires so does the other and the temporal relationship between the two firings is very constant. In MG, because the neuromuscular junction is sick at times messages do not get across, causing one of the fascicules not to fire, thus demonstrating conduction block. Jitter is delayed firing, which occurs because in MG more acetylcholine may be required to initiate firing than usual, so there may be a delay while more is diffusing across the neuromuscular junction. In purely ocular MG there are often no electrophysiological abnormalities demonstrable in the limbs. Single fibre EMG of orbicularis oculi is then helpful. A test that is now falling out of favour is the Tensilon test. A small amount of a short-acting acetylcholine esterase inhibitor (Tensilon, edrophonium) is injected intravenously. If there is a neuromuscular transmission defect the transient rise in the amount of acetylcholine available will result in transient improvement. Clinical diplopia or a ptosis will improve for a minute or two. The test is not without hazard and requires pretreatment with atropine and cardiopulmonary resuscitation to be available. In addition both false positives and false negatives are not uncommon.

Initial treatment may well be with longer lasting acetylcholine esterase inhibitors such as Mestinon (pyridostigmine), though these are limited in their usefulness, both because they are not very effective in severe MG and because of gastrointestinal side effects. The latter may be ameliorated with anticholinergics (e.g. atropine). More definitive treatment needs to be directed at the immune response. Both corticosteroids and azathioprine are used in the long-term management. Initially, patients can deteriorate when being started on steroids and plasma exchange is a useful and rapidly effective short-term measure. In the younger patients thymectomy may be curative. In older patients thymectomy is usually indicated if a thymoma is present, but paradoxically it does not help the MG. Patients with an underlying thymoma often have antistriated muscle antibodies as well as anti-acetylcholine receptor antibodies.

Lambert–Eaton myasthenic syndrome (LEMS)

This is such a rare condition that it only deserves a mention because of its neurophysiological neatness. In LEMS antibodies are directed against the calcium channel on the presynaptic membrane of the neuromuscular junction. This results in difficulties in releasing acetylcholine vesicles, producing weakness. As more depolarizations in a train of impulses arrive presynaptic intracellular calcium tends to rise, thus overcoming the problem. This leads to increased strength on activity and electrophysiologically an increment on a repetitive stimulation test. Deep tendon reflexes are reduced or absent, but become stronger after exercise. About half the patients with LEMS have an underlying small cell lung cancer.

Botulism

This is caused by the exotoxin of *Clostridium botulinum*. In adults it is usually caused by eating foodstuffs that have been contaminated by the heat resistant spores which have subsequently germinated and produced toxin. Infection of wounds can result in systemic spread of the toxin. Particularly in infants up to 6 months of age the gastrointestinal tract can become colonized with *Clostridium botulinum* with subsequent toxin production. Symptoms appear from 12 to 48 hours after ingestion of the toxin. A rapidly progressive paralysis develops. The deep tendon reflexes are retained. As the toxin irreversibly binds to the presynaptic region of the neuromuscular junction recovery takes days to months. Patients often require prolonged ventilatory support.

Neuromuscular blocking agents

In modern anaesthesia there are usually two aspects to the process. The first is to reduce conscious level, hopefully to a point where there is no recollection (though there has been interesting work on the effect of audiotaped messages given during operations). The second is muscle relaxation to allow the surgeon to do their worst. Frequently, neuromuscular blocking agents are used, such as suxamethonium, which bind to the acetylcholine receptors. If a patient has subclinical myasthenia gravis and is given one of these agents then paralysis is prolonged, sometimes for days, and the patient will require respiratory support. A deficiency of pseudocholinesterase can also cause prolonged weakness and apnoea after depolarizing relaxants have been administered. An additional neuromuscular anaesthetic hazard is malignant hyperpyrexia which is a dominantly inherited susceptibility to halothane or suxamethonium in particular, though any anaesthetic agent can precipitate an attack. Hyperpyrexia and muscle stiffness develops. Treatment is with dantrolene. The condition has some similarities with neuroleptic malignant syndrome (see Chapter 19).

Muscular disease

There are three types of muscle diseases, the dystrophies, myositises and myopathies. The dystrophies are genetic in origin and usually present in childhood. The myositises are due to an inflammation in muscle. Proximal muscles are usually affected predominantly and there is muscle tenderness. The myopathies are due to hormonal or biochemical problems and again predominantly affect the proximal musculature, but without tenderness.

Muscular dystrophies

This group of disorders are inherited degenerations of muscle, usually presenting in childhood. I have mentioned only the more important ones.

Duchenne muscular dystrophy
This is an X-linked recessive disorder with an incidence of 1/3500 live born boys. Very rarely girls can be affected and female carriers may have minor symptoms. Towards the end of the third year of life there is difficulty walking, falling and climbing stairs. Ninety per cent develop pseudohypertrophy of the calf muscles. Most patients are unable to walk by the age of 10 years. Death usually occurs towards the end of the second decade. The gene has been identified and is responsible for the production of a large protein called dystrophin which has an important structural role in muscle. Genetic means of detecting female carriers are imperfect, but muscle biopsy abnormalities in dystrophin staining and immunoblot analysis are currently the best techniques for carrier detection.

Becker muscular dystrophy
This is also due to a mutation of the dystrophin gene and together with Duchenne muscular dystrophy these conditions are sometimes called Xp21 muscular dystrophy. Onset is between the ages of 5 and 25. There is gradual weakness and wasting of the pelvic and pectoral muscles with patients unable to walk 25 years or more after onset.

Dystrophia myotonica
This is an ideal condition for finals examinations, in that it is rare, has good physical signs and is only slowly progressive, so patients can be used year after year. It is an autosomal dominant disorder with an incidence of 13.5/10 000 live births. The most characteristic feature of the disease is myotonia, which is a failure of muscle to relax after contraction. This can be demonstrated in patients by asking them to open and close their hands rapidly, or by striking the thenar eminence with a patellae hammer and observing the slow relaxation of the thumb back to its usual position. Sometimes a dimple in the muscle can be seen where it has been struck that is slow to fill. In addition to myotonia there is muscular weakness and atrophy. The disorder is a diffuse systemic problem and is associated with cataracts, frontal balding in males, gonadal atrophy, cardiomyopathy, hypersomnia, diabetes and intellectual impairment. Patients have a typical facial appearance of a thin hatchet face with bilateral ptosis and frontal balding. The condition often presents between the ages of 20 and 50. Severe disability occurs 15 to 20 years after onset. Not infrequently the disorder is diagnosed in the mother when a floppy baby is born. The genetic abnormality is an abnormal CGT repeat within the protein kinase gene on chromosome 19q13. Part of the explanation for the severe infantile form seen in babies born to mothers with dystrophica myotonica may be 'anticipation' where the number of abnormal repeats increases with each subsequent generation.

The inflammatory myositises – polymyositis, dermatomyositis and inclusion-body myositis (Table 14.2)

The incidence of polymyositis, dermatomyositis and inclusion-body myositis is about 1/100 000. The weakness is proximal and slowly progressive (weeks to months, inclusion-body myositis may progress over years). Fine movements are only involved late in polymyositis and dermatomyositis but early in inclusion-body myositis. Dysphagia and difficulty holding up the head are common while

	Dermatomyositis	Polymyositis	Inclusion-body myositis
Muscles involved	Proximal	Proximal	Distal
Biopsy	Vessels involved	Muscle	Inclusion bodies
Immune attack	Humoral	T-cell	T-cell
Associations	Skin and malignancy	Drugs	None
Treatment	Steroids and azathioprine	Steroids and azathioprine	None

Table 14.2 Summary of the inflammatory myositises

ocular muscles remain normal. As well as muscle weakness dermatological changes are seen in dermatomyositis with a heliotrope rash on the upper eyelids, a flat red rash on the face and upper trunk and erythema of the knuckles. Dermatomyositis may occur with systemic sclerosis, mixed connective tissue disease and other autoimmune conditions and is associated with an increased incidence of underlying malignancy. Polymyositis may be in association with systemic autoimmune or connective tissue diseases. A similar condition can be precipitated by penicillamine and zidovudine.

Extramuscular systems can be involved with systemic symptoms such as fever, malaise and weight loss. The heart and lungs are frequently involved.

Muscle biopsy is the definitive test. In polymyositis the inflammatory attack appears to be centred on muscle itself while in dermatomyositis it appears to be directed at the blood vessels in muscle. In inclusion-body myositis as well as general signs of inflammation in muscle there are basophilic granular inclusions distributed around the edge of slit-like vacuoles and eosinophilic cytoplasmic inclusions. On electron microscopy granules containing membranous whorls are seen. The autoimmune response in dermatomyositis is primarily humoral while in polymyositis and inclusion-body myositis it is T-cell mediated.

First line therapy for polymyositis and dermatomyositis is prednisolone, 1 mg/kg per day for 3–4 weeks, tapering to an alternate day regimen. Azathioprine, up to 3 mg/kg/day, is used as a steroid sparing agent. Patients with interstitial lung disease have a high mortality

and require cyclophosphamide. Inclusion body myositis is generally resistant to all therapies.

Polymyalgia rheumatica
This is a condition of the elderly which is associated with temporal arteritis. It presents with pain in the muscles, local tenderness and minor constitutional upset. Muscle biopsy and creatinine kinase levels are usually normal though the ESR is elevated. The condition responds magically to steroids.

Myopathies

Myopathies are usually due to hormonal disturbances or biochemical abnormalities, but life is never quite as simple as it first appears. While muscular dystrophies are genetically determined and appear in childhood some myopathies, while being biochemically medicated, are genetically determined and can appear in childhood. The distinction is more about common usage than semantic absolutes.

Endocrine myopathies
The two most common are steroid and thyroid hormone associated. Steroid myopathy can occur in Cushing's disease, but it is much more common as an iatrogenic product of steroid therapy. It usually takes several weeks to appear, but has been seen as an acute myositis after megadoses of methylprednisolone. The weakness is proximal and not tender. It resolves on stopping the steroids. In thyrotoxicosis there is also a proximal myopathy. As there can be fasciculations this can be confused with motor neurone disease

(see Chapter 20). Hypothyroidism, acromegaly, hypopituitarism, and osteomalacia have also been reported to be associated with myopathies.

Metabolic myopathies – acquired
A myopathy can be seen in renal failure. Sometimes it is attributable to concomitant osteomalacia, but in other patients it seems directly attributable to the uraemia.

Metabolic myopathies – genetic
GLYCOGEN STORAGE DISEASE
The two most important glycogen storage diseases are McArdle's disease and acid maltase deficiency. *McArdle's disease* is due to a myophosphorylase deficiency. It is inherited in an autosomal recessive fashion and presents with generalized muscular pain and stiffness that increases on exercise. *Acid maltase deficiency* is again autosomal recessive. It can present in childhood or adulthood in varying severity. Not uncommonly it presents with proximal weakness and respiratory failure.

Mitochondrial myopathies
In recent years the importance of the mitochondria and their associated disorders has been appreciated. These conditions are certainly a lot more common than was previously supposed. Defects in mitochondrial function

result in energy deficient states in cells. Some mitochondrial proteins are encoded on mitochondrial DNA. Mitochondrial DNA is inherited from the mother, resulting in maternal transmission of these disorders. Which particular syndrome is manifest will depend on how many defective mitochondria are present in which particular tissue. The various syndromes are given in Table 14.3 for reference.

Chronic **P**rogressive **E**xternal **O**phthalmoplegia
Leber's hereditary optic neuropathy
Kearns–Sayre syndrome
  ocular myopathy
  retinal pigmentation
  cerebellar degeneration
  cardiomyopathy
MELAS syndrome
  Mitochondrial
  Encephalomyelopathy
  Lactic **A**cidosis
  Stroke-like episodes
MERRF
  Mitochondrial myopathy
  myoclonic **E**pilepsy
  Ragged-**R**ed **F**ibres (on muscle biopsy)
Additional findings
  dementia
  deafness
  seizures

Table 14.3 The mitochondrial syndromes

MCQs for Chapter 14

The MCQs are either true T or false F. The answers are given in Appendix 3. Negatively mark your answers; a point for a correct answer, deduct a point for an incorrect response. If you score 24 or more you pass.

1. **In myasthenia gravis:**
   A The hallmark of myasthenia gravis is fatiguability.
   B Respiratory muscles are usually the first to be affected.
   C Thymoma is more common in older patients.
   D The Tensilon test is very sensitive and specific.

2. **Lambert–Eaton myasthenic syndrome (LEMS) and botulism:**
   A In LEMS antibodies are directed against the subunit of the acetylcholine receptor.
   B About half of the patients with LEMS will have an underlying small cell lung cancer.
   C Botulism is caused by *Clostridium difficile*.
   D Recovery from botulism takes months.

3.
   A Suxamethonium binds to acetylcholine receptors.
   B Pseudocholinesterase deficiency is a cause of prolonged apnoea after anaesthesia.
   C Malignant hyperpyrexia can be precipitated by diazepam.
   D Myasthenia gravis is not affected by neuromuscular blocking agents.

4. **Muscular dystrophies:**
   A Duchenne muscular dystrophy is an X-linked recessive disorder.
   B In Duchenne muscular dystrophy onset is in early adulthood.
   C Carriers of Duchenne can be detected by dystrophin staining.
   D Becker muscular dystrophy is a more severe form of Duchenne muscular dystrophy.

5. **Dystrophia myotonica is associated with:**
   A Frontal balding.
   B Diabetes.
   C Cataracts.
   D Achlorhydria.

6. **Polymyositis:**
   A Initially affects the distal musculature.
   B May be associated with systemic auto-immune disease.
   C Is humorally mediated.
   D On muscle biopsy basophilic granular inclusions are seen round vacuoles.

7. **Dermatomyositis:**
   A Is associated with a heliotrope rash.
   B Biopsy shows blood vessel involvement.
   C Is not associated with malignancy.
   D Is unresponsive to treatment.

8. **Inclusion-body myositis and polymyalgia rheumatica:**
   A Inclusion-body myositis involves fine movements early.
   B Inclusion-body myositis responds well to plasmaphaeresis.
   C Polymyalgia rheumatica is associated with a high ESR.
   D Polymyalgia rheumatica is classically a condition of adolescents.

9. **Myopathies:**
   A Steroid administration is associated with a distal myopathy.
   B In thyrotoxicosis fasciculations may be seen.
   C McArdle's disease may present with muscle pain and stiffness.
   D Acid maltase deficiency is inherited in an autosomal dominant fashion.

10. **Mitochondrial disorders are associated with:**
    A Cardiomyopathy.
    B Pancreatitis.
    C Myoclonic epilepsy.
    D Myoglobinaemia.

15. Cerebrovascular disease

Objectives

The aim of this chapter is to discuss the cerebrovascular diseases. Topics addressed are:

- Risk factors
- Assessment of a patient with a 'stroke'
- TIA
- Multi-infarct dementia
- Dissection
- Binswanger's encephalopathy
- Cerebral vasculitis
- Intracerebral haemorrhage
- Subarachnoid haemorrhage
- Arteriovenous malformations
- Venous sinus thrombosis

Basic science – lipids

Traditionally the cerebrovascular diseases have been a Cinderella subspecialty of the neurosciences. However, it is the third most important cause of death in Western countries and fills 7% of hospital beds. Survivors place great burdens on the community, both financially, physically and emotionally. The co-occurrence of academic interest, political will and effective strategies for management and treatment has led to a nascence of activity in this area.

A stroke is a complex symptom resulting from intracerebral haemorrhage or from embolism or thrombosis of the cerebral vessels. It implies a sudden event. The term is of historical interest, but is not a diagnosis. It comes from the idea that a cerebrovascular accident is a stroke from the hand of God. As clinicians our diagnosis should be more precise.

The differential diagnosis of 'stroke' is given in Table 15.1. The purpose of that table is not that it should be memorized, but as a reminder that there is a differential diagnosis of stroke.

Risk factors

The major risk factors for cerebrovascular disease are given in Table 15.2.

The assessment of a patient with a cerebrovascular event

In North America cerebrovascular events have been renamed 'brain attacks' in order to impress on both lay and medical persons the importance and urgency of the situation.

When assessing a patient with a brain

HAEMORRHAGE
Subarachnoid haemorrhage
Intracerebral haemorrhage
  Hypertensive
  AVM
  Aneurysm
  Vasculitis, e.g. amyloid angiopathy
  Haemorrhage into a tumour
INFARCT (a localized or circumscribed area of ischaemic
  tissue necrosis due to inadequate blood flow)
Hypoperfusion
  Shock, e.g.
    MI
    Sepsis
    Bleeding
    PE
    Hypovolaemia
    Cardiac surgery
  Tight stenosis proximal in arterial tree
  Dissection
Thrombus – Virchow's triad
  Stasis or low flow (after a stenosis)
  Damage to vessel walls
    Atheroma
    Vasculitis
    Temporal arteritis
    Isolated angitis of the CNS
    Meningitis – bacterial, TB, syphilis
    Fibrinoid degeneration
    Dissection
  Alteration in coagulability of blood
    Hyperviscosity – polycythaemia
    Coagulability
      Lupus anticoagulant
      Low antithrombin III or protein C or S
Embolus
  Hyperviscosity and hypercoagulability
  Heart
    Foramen ovale
    Valve
      Rheumatic fever
      Prosthetic
      Infective
    Left atrium and ventricle
    Rhythm, especially atrial fibrillation
  Proximal in arterial tree – atheroma at bifurcation

Table 15.1 Differential diagnosis of a 'stroke'

Age – incidence rises sharply over 60
Hypertension
Cardiac disease
Extracranial vascular disease, e.g. carotid atheroma
Diabetes mellitus
Hyperlipidaemia
Packed cell volume >0.5
Smoking – increases risk ×3
Oral contraceptive pill and pregnancy
Crack and cocaine

Table 15.2 Risk factors for cerebrovascular disease

attack a few simple questions need to be addressed.

1. Is it an infarct or a haemorrhage?

Clinically it is impossible to be certain, but there are various clues set out in Table 15.3. A CT scan is needed for certainty.

2. If it is an infarct what sort is it?

There are two aspects to this question. The first is about embolism versus thrombosis. Again, clinically it is difficult to be certain, but the presence of valvular disease or atrial fibrillation is circumstantial evidence for embolism. The second part of this question relates to the vascular territory involved. Bamford's classification (Table 15.4) is both practical and useful. The neuroanatomy is discussed in Chapter 9.

TACI implies either a near complete middle cerebral artery infarct or a carotid artery occlusion with both middle and anterior cerebral artery territory infarction. The patient is drowsy with a dense hemiplegia, eyes deviated to the side of the infarction, with a severe global aphasia if dominant hemisphere is affected, or visuospatial neglect and denial of illness if non-dominant hemisphere.

PACI is usually an infarction in the territory of a branch of the middle cerebral artery and involves some cortical functions, but is short of a TACI. An example of a PACI is seen on the CT in Fig. 15.1 where there is a well-defined infarct in the right middle cerebral artery territory, but only involving the anterior part.

A POCI is an infarct in the vertebrobasilar territory, including the posterior cerebral arteries. There will usually be nausea and vomiting in conjunction with brain stem signs. Not infrequently there is an occipital headache.

There are four main lacunar syndromes recognized which allows a diagnosis of a LACI to be made, they are:

Symptom	Bleed	Infarct
Loss of consciousness	At presentation	Unusual
Headache	The rule	Occasionally
Nausea and vomiting	Frequent	Posterior fossa
Coma	Frequent	Late if at all
Signs of herniation	Often	Late (24–48 hr)
Stuttering course	Rarely	Frequent
Previous TIAs	Very unusual	Sometimes

Table 15.3 Bleed vs Infarct 'Anything can be anything'

Total **A**nterior **C**erebral **I**nfarction
Partial **A**nterior **C**erebral **I**nfarction
POsterior **C**irculation **I**nfarct
LACunar **I**nfarct

Table 15.4 Bamford's classification of cerebral infarcts

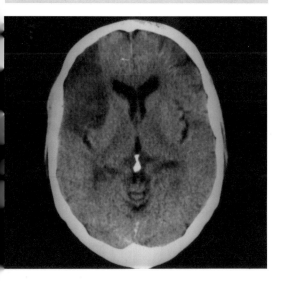

Fig. 15.1 An example of a partial anterior cerebral infarct (PACI).

1. Pure motor hemiparesis
2. Pure hemisensory disturbance
3. Hemisensorimotor disturbance
4. Ataxic hemiparesis.

3. What needs to be done in terms of acute management?

The key areas of acute management are blood pressure control, hydration, infection and glycemic control. In cerebral infarction, unless the diastolic blood pressure is over 130 mmHg, it is better to allow blood pressure to settle of its own accord as precipitous falls will reduce perfusion pressure. If the patient is shocked then the blood pressure will have to be increased, either with fluids or pressors. If swallowing or consciousness is impaired then in the first instance hydration should be via an intravenous line. Allowing the patient to dehydrate for 48 hours and then see if they need a nasogastric tube seems barbaric. Most people would be feeling unwell after 48 hours of fluid deprivation and a time of cerebral infarction is not the moment for haemoconcentration. The only caveat to this is that early mortality in large strokes will be due to cerebral oedema and one could argue that some mild fluid restriction would be appropriate if cerebral oedema is developing (1.5–2 l/day). A fever is a good way of increasing the metabolic rate of tissues and should be avoided while brain tissues are partially ischaemic. So prompt treatment of infection and use of paracetamol to reduce fever is important. Elevated blood glucose is another way of increasing infarct size so good glycaemic control is essential. In cerebellar infarction hydrocephalus and brain-stem compression can develop, requiring neurosurgical intervention. Thrombolysis for infarcts presenting within 3 hours has become routine practice in the USA, but is currently not used in the UK. Neuroprotective agents may soon become a routine part of the management of cerebral infarction.

Case history

Mrs Burslem is a 65-year-old retired cup sponger who was found by her husband, when he returned from walking the dog, on the floor of their living room unable to speak or get up. She was taken to hospital and found to have a dense right hemiparesis, she was mute with a receptive component to her aphasia. She had visuospatial neglect to the right and a probable right homonymous hemianopsia. A clinical diagnosis of a TACI was made and as she was assessed within 6 hours of the event her family was offered the opportunity of enrolling her in a phase III trial of a neuroprotective agent. She received either placebo or active agent by intravenous infusion and had a CT scan of the head, which was essentially normal.

The next day on the ward she was able to say yes and no and her comprehension had much improved. The field deficit and visuospatial neglect had disappeared, but she remained with a dense homonymous hemianopsia. A repeat CT scan at 1 week showed patchy hypodensity within the distribution of the left middle cerebral artery. Prior to her cerebral infarction she had smoked 20 cigarettes a day. She was found to have a cholesterol of 7.1 mmol/l, a triglyceride of 2.3 mmol/l and an HDL of only 0.9 mmol/l. She required nasogastric feeding and after 2 weeks a percutaneous gastrostomy tube was inserted. Reasonable power returned to her right leg, but the hand remained plegic. After 6 weeks on the neurology ward she was transferred to a rehabilitation ward for a further 6 weeks' rehabilitation prior to discharge home. At that point she was able to swallow, so had had the gastrostomy tube removed, she was able to make conversation, though this was slow and laboured and she was able to walk 10 metres.

Routine	In selected patients
Non-contrast CT of the head	Carotid Dopplers
ECG	Protein S&C
CXR	Sickle cell
FBC	Antithrombin III
ESR	Anti–phospholipid antibodies
U&E	Echocardiogram
Glucose	24-hour ECG
Fasting lipids and cholesterol	MRI
VDRL	Cerebral angiography

Table 15.5 Investigations to be considered in cerebral infarction and TIA

4. What needs to be done for secondary prevention?

The risk factors for cerebrovascular disease (see Table 15.2) need to be identified and long-term strategies for their amelioration need to be enacted. The simplest are blood pressure control, cessation of smoking and an aspirin a day. A list of investigations to be considered is given in Table 15.5. Atherosclerotic cerebral ischaemia is the same disease as coronary atherosclerosis, the difference being only the organ involved. The same risk factors are involved and the same strategies for control should be employed. Recovering from the stroke and succumbing to a heart attack 5 years later is a significant failure of secondary prevention. Aggressive management of hyperlipidaemia is an important part of any secondary prevention programme. Patients with PACIs need to have their carotid arteries assessed for stenosis as surgery would be appropriate if a stenosis of greater than 70% was found on the side of the infarction.

Transient ischaemic attack (TIA)

A transient ischaemic attack is an episode of focal cerebral ischaemia whose symptoms last for less than 24 hours. A TIA can occur in the eye causing transient unilateral visual loss and this is called amaurosis fugax. Usually a TIA will last less than an hour. About one in five TIA victims will have a completed stroke in the subsequent 5 years; however, a similar number will have a myocardial infarction. As well as addressing the risk factors for CVA (Table 15.2) and starting patients on an

Basic science – lipids

The importance and complexity of hyperlipidaemia is now being appreciated. High levels of cholesterol, LDL (low-density lipoprotein) and triglyceride are associated with atherosclerotic disease, whereas HDL (high-density lipoprotein) has an inverse relationship with atherogenesis. On average each person in the UK takes in 120 g of triglyceride and 500 mg of cholesterol a day. In the gut this is packaged into triglyceride rich chylomicrons which reach the blood stream via the thoracic duct. They are hydrolysed by lipoprotein lipase releasing triglyceride. This is in turn broken down into free fatty acids to provide energy. Cholesterol is essential for cell membranes, myelin sheaths and steroid hormones.

Most cells can synthesize cholesterol from acetate. Hydroxymethylglutaryl coenzyme A reductase limits cholesterol biosynthesis. In the fasting state endogenous cholesterol and triglyceride are transported by VLDL (very low-density lipoproteins). Lipoprotein lipase hydrolyses these to LDL. LDL is catabolized in the liver. It is taken up by a high affinity receptor mechanism and by scavenger pathways. In heterozygous familial hypercholesterolaemia only about half the normal receptor activity is present. In the more severe but rarer homozygous form there are no LDL receptors. When excess LDL is present it may pass through the endothelium into the subendothelial space where monocytes are attracted. They try to scavenge the LDL and become fat laden foam cells which are unable to migrate. They accumulate, breaching the endothelium layer, forming a fatty streak which is the basis of an atheromatous plaque. HDL has a role in transporting cholesterol to the liver for catabolism.

The initial approach to the management of hyperlipidaemia is control of dietary intake of lipids and weight reduction. Secondary hyperlipidaemia due to causes such as diabetes or drugs (thiazides and β-blockers) needs to be excluded.

However, diet alone will prove inadequate in many patients. Fortunately there are well tolerated and effective drugs now available for lipid lowering. The need for long-term medical treatment will depend on the level of the fasting lipids and the presence of other risk factors.

Resins and statins are used as first line medications for hypercholesterolaemia while fibrates are used when the triglyceride is elevated as well as the cholesterol. A statin has been demonstrated to lower the frequency of subsequent coronary events in patients with average cholesterol levels who have had a myocardial infarction.

aspirin a day (75–300 mg) for its antiplatelet effect, patients with carotid territory TIA (including amaurosis fugax) should have their carotids imaged. Initially carotid ultrasound can be used to detect a stenosis. If there is a 50% or greater stenosis MR angiography or spiral CT angiography can give accurate measurements of the degree of stenosis. There is controversy over the need to proceed to conventional angiography as it carries a 1–3% risk of stroke. Complete occlusion is not an indication for carotid endarterectomy. As it can be difficult to differentiate a tight stenosis from occlusion a conventional angiogram may be necessary. In greater than 70% stenosed carotid endarterectomy reduces the risks of a subsequent stroke on that side. The reduction in risk and the risk of the investigations and surgical procedures themselves are finely balanced and the advisability of proceeding will largely depend on the competence of the surgical team, balance of risk factors in the individual patient and the patient's personal preference.

Multi-infarct dementia

The second most common form of dementia and probably the most preventable is multi-infarct dementia. If enough of the brain is damaged one must end up demented. However, the situation is slightly more complex in that infarcts in the dominant hemisphere are more likely to lead to intellectual impairment; though this could be because we assess cognitive status almost exclusively through the medium of language. In addition a large number of patients with multiple cerebral infarcts and dementia have other pathologies such as Alzheimer's disease present. It is probably much easier to dement if there is more than one process heading in that direction (the double hit theory). Patients with atrial fibrillation who are unanticoagulated, poorly controlled hypertensives and smokers, who are having multiple infarcts are obviously target groups in whom intervention might help prevent the development of multi-infarct dementia.

Dissection

The carotid, vertebral and intracerebral arteries can all dissect, causing cerebral ischaemia. While a rare cause of cerebral infarction it should be considered in younger patients, particularly if there is pain in the neck. Classically, carotid dissection follows a blow to the neck, but can be spontaneous. Anticoagulants can help to prevent embolic complications but their role is controversial.

Binswanger's encephalopathy

I mention this condition mostly because of the sound of its name. In hypertensive patients the small perforating arterioles become involved in hyaline degeneration. This results in ischaemia to the white matter. Individual infarcts can result in lacunar syndromes, but *en masse* this results in Binswanger's encephalopathy. There are generalized ischaemic changes diffusely in the white matter. On the CT this can be seen as hypodensity around the ventricles. On T2 MR the periventricular area is hyperintense. Clinically it can be asymptomatic or present with a dementia or gait apraxia.

Cerebral vasculitis

While the most common cause of cerebral ischaemia is atherosclerosis, either via thrombosis or embolism, the cerebral vasculitises are

Temporal (giant cell) arteritis
Takayasu's disease
Systemic vasculitis
Rheumatoid disease
Wegener's granulomatosis
Behçet's disease
Isolated angitis of the central nervous system
(Systemic lupus erythematosus [antiphospholipid syndrome])*

*Lupus very rarely, if ever, causes a true vasculitis, but does cause cerebral ischaemia.

Table 15.6 Inflammatory vascular disorders causing cerebral ischaemia

an important treatable cause of cerebral ischaemia. They are given in Table 15.6.

Temporal arteritis

This is the only relatively common cerebral vasculitis. It occurs in patients over 50 years of age. The patients have usually been feeling constitutionally unwell for a few weeks. They develop a tenderness of the scalp, particularly around the temporal areas. Lying the head on a pillow is sore as is combing the hair. Chewing can be painful because of jaw claudication. Because there is a vasculitis occlusion of blood vessels in the head occurs. This can result in sudden unilateral loss of vision, diplopia or evidence of cerebral ischaemia. The ESR is usually over 50 mm/h. A temporal artery biopsy may show the vasculitis. If suspected then the patient should be given 60 mg of prednisolone immediately, as there is a danger of permanent visual loss. It is very rare for temporal arteritis not to be associated with an elevated ESR. The biopsy should be done within 48 hours of initiating the steroids, but with a good history and elevated ESR a negative biopsy should not change the diagnosis. There is a magical response to steroids and if the patient does not think you are God's gift to the medical profession within 24 hours then the diagnosis is in doubt. Unfortunately, steroids have a non-specific effect on aches and pains, somewhat confusing the issue. The steroids can be reduced over the next month to 30 mg a day and then gradually reduced over the next year or two, depending on the patient's symptoms and their ESR.

Intracerebral haemorrhage

Intracranial haemorrhages are usually into the subarachnoid space, intraparenchymal or both. If the nidus of the haemorrhage is within the parenchyma then hypertension is the most common cause, but arteriovenous malformations, neoplasms, vasculitis and amyloid angiopathy are other causes. Subarachnoid haemorrhages are usually caused by berry aneurysms, but can be idiopathic, due to arteriovenous malformations or blood dyscrasias.

Hypertensive bleeds

Hypertensive bleeds occur where there are perforating arterioles. The small blood vessels undergo hyaline degeneration secondary to elevated blood pressure. This can either result in lacunar infarction or small aneurysm formation which can burst, allowing blood to pour out into the brain's substance. The most common locations and signs are given in Table 15.7. Intracranial haemorrhages are associated with signs of raised intracranial pressure (headache, vomiting, clouding of consciousness, false localizing signs and possibly papilloedema).

Neurosurgical intervention is sometimes important in younger patients with a non-dominant hemisphere haemorrhage who are in danger of herniating and in cerebellar haemorrhages where the brain stem is being compressed.

Amyloid angiopathy

Up to 10% of intracerebral haemorrhages are due to this condition. It is particularly likely to be present if haemorrhages occur in locations other than those seen in hypertension and if haemorrhages are recurrent. Amyloid is deposited in the cerebral vasculature resulting in fragile vessels. It can be inherited in an autosomal dominant fashion. The natural history is of recurrent haemorrhages and cerebral ischaemia resulting in progressive neurological disability and death.

Subarachnoid haemorrhage (SAH)

Any patient presenting with sudden onset of severe headache has had a subarachnoid haemorrhage until proven otherwise. Other associated features are nausea, presyncope or loss of consciousness, photophobia, neck stiffness and focal neurological signs or symptoms. It may be precipitated by physical exertion, often coitus. It is caused by blood rushing out into the subarachnoid space and is a cause of sudden death. The patients who come to medical attention have stopped bleeding, so concern should be focused on stopping the next bleed and dealing with the consequences of the current one. The initial investigation is a CT scan of the head. If this is performed within 48 hours of the event it will demonstrate an SAH in over 80% of cases. However, if it is negative the patient will have to undergo a lumbar puncture. The abnormalities sought will be an elevated pressure, a raised red cell count, often with a white cell pleocytosis due to the meningeal reaction, and the presence of xanthochromia. Xanthochromia is the pigmentary change in CSF due to the breakdown of red cells. It is useful when one

Location	Signs
Basal ganglia	Hemiparesis
Pons	Pin-point pupils and oculomotor dysfunction
	Long track signs
Cerebellum	Ataxia
	Nystagmus
	Vomiting

Table 15.7 Locations and signs of the common hypertensive haemorrhages

has a bloody tap and it is not clear if it was traumatic or not. In addition it can suggest an SAH up to 3 weeks after the event when the excess of red cells have cleared. Xanthochromia can be detectable to the naked eye, but a photospectroscopic examination is more sensitive. Because it takes about 6 hours to develop, and one can never be certain a tap is not traumatic, the lumbar puncture should be deferred until about 12 hours after the event.

Once an SAH has been diagnosed the cerebral vasculature will require imaging. Currently this is done with intra-arterial contrast agents and X-rays, though MRI, if the resolution of MR angiography improves, will become the method of choice. Having identified the cause of the SAH surgical treatment or embolization is usually appropriate. In the period between presentation and surgery the patient's care is important. Unless the patient is comatose or showing signs of focal cerebral ischaemia the blood pressure should be kept low. A dose of 50–100 mg of atenolol (a beta blocker) a day is often appropriate. In addition, within the first 3 days nimodipine (a calcium channel blocker) should be introduced. It lowers the mortality and morbidity from SAH though the exact mechanism is uncertain. Strict rules about total bed rest are being relaxed, but patients should be kept quiet and 2 mg of diazepam three times a day is often a kindness.

There are a number of causes of SAH (Table 15.8). One problematic group are those whose angiogram is negative. In those cases where the blood on the initial CT scan was around the mid-brain there is evidence that they have a good prognosis and are likely not to have a recurrence. Those with blood in classical places for berry aneurysms (Sylvian fissures, anterior interhemispheric fissure) have an appreciable re-bleed rate from aneurysms missed on the first angiogram, so repeated angiography at a later date is justified. Some of the group of angiogram-negative patients are now being demonstrated to have cavernous haemangiomas on MRI.

Berry aneurysms

Berry aneurysms are small out-pouchings of

| Berry aneurysm |
| Arteriovenous malformations |
| Angiogram-negative (perimesencephalic venous bleeds) |
| Anticoagulants and blood dyscrasias |
| Dissecting aneurysms |
| Mycotic aneurysms |
| Traumatic |

Table 15.8 Causes of subarachnoid haemorrhage

the arterial wall that usually occur at the bifurcation of arteries. They are the most common cause of SAH. The most common sites for berry aneurysms are around the circle of Willis, particularly on the anterior communicating artery, at the bifurcation of the middle cerebral artery, and at the top of the carotid. A posterior communicating artery aneurysm can present with a painful third nerve palsy because of its location. Berry aneurysms can be familial in polycystic kidney disease and various other rare connective tissue disorders. If discovered, these aneurysms are usually surgically clipped, though the posterior fossa aneurysms, because of their difficult location, are frequently being treated by coil embolization.

Arteriovenous malformations

Arteriovenous malformations are the second most likely identifiable cause of SAH. As well as presenting with SAH they can present with epilepsy, focal neurological deficits or migraine. They are a congenital shortcut between the arterial and venous sides of the circulation, bypassing the capillary bed. They tend to grow as the years pass. Therapeutic options are surgical, embolization, or if they are small, radiosurgery can be effective.

Venous sinus thrombosis

Clots can occur within the venous system of the brain, most commonly the sagittal sinus. This results in venous hypertension back upstream and this can interfere with CSF absorption resulting in a picture not dissimilar to benign intracranial hypertension (see Chapter 19). Venous infarcts and haemorrhages can also occur. The diagnosis is usually made with MRI or the venous phase of angiography.

Venous sinus thrombosis is often idiopathic, but pregnancy, infection, Behçet's disease, lupus and other hypercoagulable states are causes. Treatment is usually with anticoagulation, even when haemorrhage is present.

MCQs for Chapter 15

The MCQs are either true T or false F. The answers are given in Appendix 3. Negatively mark your answers; a point for a correct answer, deduct a point for an incorrect response. If you score 24 or more you pass.

1. **Risk factors for stroke include:**
   A Smoking.
   B Pregnancy.
   C Hypothyroidism.
   D Bronchiectasis.

2. **Causes of intracerebral haemorrhage include:**
   A Hypertension.
   B Amyloid angiopathy.
   C Hypoperfusion.
   D Polycythaemia.

3. **Factors in favour of intracerebral haemorrhage versus infarct are:**
   A A stuttering course.
   B Previous TIAs.
   C Loss of consciousness at presentation.
   D Headache.

4. **Features of total anterior cerebral infarction include:**
   A Nystagmus.
   B Dense hemiplegia.
   C Eyes deviated away from the side of the infarct.
   D Visuospatial neglect.

5. **Lacunar syndromes include:**
   A Pure motor hemiparesis.
   B Isolated aphasia.
   C Hemisensory disturbance.
   D Dysarthria and nystagmus.

6. **Routine investigations in presumed cerebral infarction include:**
   A Non-contrast CT of the head.
   B Carotid Doppler.
   C ECG.
   D Antiphospholipid antibodies.

7. **Multi-infarct dementia:**
   A Is the most common form of dementia.
   B Is associated with hypertension.
   C Is associated with atrial fibrillation.
   D Is primarily due to lesions in the non-dominant hemisphere.

8. **Causes of cerebral vasculitis include:**
   A Rheumatoid disease.
   B Wegener's granulomatosis.
   C Diabetes mellitus.
   D Protein S and protein C deficiency.

9. **Temporal arteritis:**
   A Usually the patient is over 50 years of age.
   B Usually the ESR is over 50 mm/h.
   C Can be excluded on temporal artery biopsy.
   D Is treated with non-steroidal anti-inflammatories.

10. **Subarachnoid haemorrhage is associated with:**
    A Coitus.
    B Sudden onset severe headache.
    C Sudden death.
    D Xanthochromia.

16. Epilepsy

Objectives

In this chapter we shall discuss the seizure disorders. We shall address:

- The definition of epilepsy
- Non-epileptic seizure disorder
- Drug treatment of epilepsy
- Surgical treatment of epilepsy
- Advice given to patients
- Prescribing for females of child-bearing age

Basic science – how AEDs work

What is epilepsy?

Epilepsy is extraordinarily difficult to define. The ninth edition of Brain (*Brain's Disease of the Nervous System* (J Walton, ed.), Oxford University Press, 1993) provides the following; 'Epilepsy is a paroxysmal and transitory disturbance of the functions of the brain which develops suddenly, ceases spontaneously, and exhibits a conspicuous tendency to recurrence', which would do for some forms of migraine. The tenth edition quotes Hughlings Jackson contribution from 1873 as being 'the name for occasional sudden, excessive, rapid and local discharges of the grey matter', but then David Chadwick goes on to say 'an epileptic seizure can be defined as an intermittent, stereotyped, disturbance of consciousness, behaviour, emotion, motor function or sensation that on clinical grounds is believed to result from cortical neuronal discharge. Epilepsy can then be defined as a condition in which seizures recur, usually spontaneously'. From these ponderings of the great and the good we can extract the following features. It is paroxysmal, recurrent, and frequently has correlates on the surface EEG. It is an electrical storm in the brain.

Epidemiology

About 1% of the population currently have epilepsy and about 3% of the population will experience a seizure during their lifetime. It is more common at either extremes of life.

Classification

The classification of the epilepsies is the key to their understanding. The medical classification has been revised and has discarded the terms 'grand mal' and 'petit mal'. The patients still use these terms, but usually in a manner completely dissimilar to the original intention. The modern classification is a mixture of pathophysiology and phenomenology (not dissimilar to medicine in general), and is given in Table 16.1. The first and most important differentiation is between attacks that start all over the brain (primarily generalized) and those that start in a focal area (focal seizures). The most common primary generalized seizures are the tonic-clonic type, which used to

Generalized
   Tonic-clonic (stiffness followed by shaking)
   Tonic
   Atonic
   Absence (*petit mal*)
   Atypical absence
   Myoclonic
Focal
   Simple
     Motor
   Complex
     Somato
     Autonomic
     Psychic
     Automatisms (has to be complex)
Partial with secondary generalization
Pseudoseizures or non-epileptic seizures

Table 16.1 The classification of seizures

Loss of consciousness
Warning
   None in primary generalized
   Stereotyped in secondary generalized, e.g. smells, fear, abnormal sensation, twitching, *déjà vu*, macropsia/micropsia
Precipitants
   Fatigue
   Flashing lights
   Ethanol withdrawal
Patient should be amnesic for the fit itself. Observers may see head turning, rolling of eyes, stiffness, rhythmical shaking, incontinence of urine, change of colour of patient
Postictally
   Confusion and disorientation
   Headache
   Aching limbs
   Drowsiness
   Sore tongue
   Wet clothes

Table 16.2 Characteristics of generalized epileptic seizures

be called grand mal, and the absence seizures, which usually occur in children and used to be called petit mal. Focal seizures are named after the phenomena they induce, which is dependent on the part of the brain where the focus is. Psychic seizures, those beginning with strange experiences such as *déjà vu*, *jamais vu*, macropsia, micropsia, are often from temporal lobe foci and are part of temporal lobe epilepsy. A focal seizure can remain localized or can begin to spread. If there is a modest amount of spread then consciousness becomes impaired. This is called complex in the classification. If the whole brain becomes involved it is called secondarily generalized.

Diagnosis

The diagnosis of epilepsy is clinical and depends on a history obtained from the patient and eye witnesses. EEG abnormalities can be supportive of a diagnosis and are useful in classifying seizure type, but on their own do not make a diagnosis. One per cent of the population have epileptiform abnormalities on their EEG without ever having epilepsy. The characteristics of primary and secondary generalized seizures are given in Table 16.2. These can be differentiated by the presence or absence of an aura or warning. In general the more bizarre and stereotyped the aura the more likely it is to be epilepsy.

Causes

Often no cause can be identified. Patients with primary generalized epilepsy are more likely to have a family history of the disorder. Presumably they have inherited a biochemical susceptibility, the leading theory being that there is something wrong with the gabaminergic system. In patients with focal epilepsies there must be something wrong with part of the brain. This may be a congenital abnormality such as a cortical malformation or an arteriovenous malformation, or may be acquired, as in post-traumatic epilepsy. In a significant number of patients with temporal lobe epilepsy there has been a prolonged seizure during childhood. This is thought to have produced sclerosis (scarring) of Ammon's horn of the hippocampus. The sclerosis then acts as a focus for seizures as the child grows up. In the older age groups the most common focal causes are cerebral ischaemia and neoplasia, both primary and secondary. Biochemical disorders such as hyponatraemia, hypoglycaemia and hypocalcinaemia have to be considered in the appropriate circumstances. Alcoholism is a frequent cause of epilepsy, both because the brain becomes damaged directly by the alcohol and by repeated trauma and because withdrawal of alcohol lowers the seizure threshold. All patients with focal seizures require an imaging study and because of the difficulty in differentiating secondarily generalized from primary generalized epilepsy all patients over 30 should have an imaging study. In children MRI should be used as it does not involve exposure to ionizing radiation.

Non-epileptic seizure disorder (pseudoseizures, hysterical or psychogenic seizures)

Non-epileptic seizure disorder (NESD) is problematic. It usually produces diagnostic difficulty, iatrogenic morbidity (and I am sure on occasion mortality) and it engenders a lot of stress in both the patient's relatives and their doctors. There is coexisting organic nervous system disease in 44%, mental retardation in 17% and concurrent epilepsy in 37%. This means that the diagnosis of a non-epileptogenic seizure does not prove that the patient has not got epilepsy. The gold standard test for diagnosing NESD is video and EEG telemetry. This involves simultaneous recording of both images, sounds and EEG so all can be compared during an attack. These facilities may

not be available and alternatives are to try to induce an attack by suggesting that one might occur while a standard EEG is being performed. The attack would have to be similar both in description and as a subjective experience with the habitual attacks for there to be any validity in concluding that the major problem is NESD. Further helpful investigations are EEG shortly after an attack as prolonged generalized epileptic seizures are often followed by slowing in the EEG and serum prolactin levels should be raised. There are some clinical pointers to the diagnosis of NESD, but none of them are absolute (Table 16.3).

Non-epileptic status is particularly hazardous as these patients fail to respond to the standard antiepileptic drugs and are therefore given more and more sedating drugs until they become respiratorally embarrassed and end up on an ITU.

Management of patients with NESD consists of providing sympathetic support without confronting the patient. As a relationship develops between the patient and the doctor there may be a tacit understanding of what is going on. It is counter-productive and incorrect to imply that patients are 'putting it on' or faking their seizures. Patients often require a sensible standard antiepileptic drug regimen because of the possibility of concurrent epileptic seizures. Sometimes patients themselves can differentiate between the two types of attacks.

Features supportive of NESD	Features supportive of epilepsy
Flailing of all four limbs	Loss of consciousness
Bilateral motor activity with preserved consciousness	Postictal period characterized by confusion, drowsiness and headache
Hip thrusting	Urinary incontinence and tongue biting
Shaking of head from side to side	Trauma
Psychosocial stressors (previous sexual abuse)	Raised serum prolactin after a convulsion
Videotape monitoring with EEG telemetry showing no seizure activity	Good response to antiepileptic drugs
Inducability without EEG correlates	Abnormal EEG

Table 16.3 Features helpful in differentiating NESD from epilepsy

Basic science – how AEDs work

To a clinician this is of little interest, but examiners live in a different universe and questions about the mechanism of action of AEDs frequently appear in the MRCP part I, despite the fact they are imperfectly understood.

GABA is the major inhibitory neurotransmitter in the CNS and potentiating its activity reduces the likelihood of seizures occurring. GABA is synthesized from glutamic acid by decarboxylation. The GABA receptor allows outflow of chloride out of the cell resulting in hyperpolarization, taking the cell membrane potential further away from the threshold. The GABA receptor has benzodiazepine and barbiturate receptor sites in close proximity which enhance the activity of the receptor. Valproate increases the synthesis and decreases the degradation of GABA. Vigabatrin is a suicidal inhibitor of GABA transaminase which is involved in its breakdown.

Glutamate and aspartate are the two major excitatory neurotransmitters in the CNS. They are involved in the initiation and spread of seizures. There are three major postsynaptic glutamate receptor types, AMPA, Quisqualate and NMDA. They are named after the ligands they preferentially bind. Lamotrigine inhibits the release of glutamate at presynaptic voltage sensitive sodium channels. While NMDA antagonists theoretically are attractive to potential AEDs they tend to result in unacceptable psychotic side effects.

Topiramate is purported to have three sites of antiepileptic action. It reduces the epileptiform discharges from voltage sensitive sodium channels. It enhances GABA at the receptor and it antagonizes the AMPA glutamate receptors.

Gabapentin was designed as a GABA analogue, but it does not bind at known GABA-minergic sites, yet still has an antiepileptic effect!

If a patient has had two or more seizures then consideration will be given to drug treatment. Over 70% of patients will be well controlled with one of the standard drugs (carbamazepine or sodium valproate). Patients should be counselled about the aims of treatment and side effects and then started on a low dose. If this does not control the attacks then the dose is gradually increased until either the attacks are controlled or symptoms of toxicity appear. Once toxicity has been reached the patient is tried on another first line drug, again gradually moving towards toxicity. If this fails the patient probably has drug-resistant epilepsy, but it is worth trying the new antiepileptics such as lamotrigine as add-ons. At some stage the diagnosis and type of epilepsy needs to be re-evaluated. Surgery and drug trials are further options to be considered by a neurologist or epileptologist at that stage. A list of the more common drugs used in epilepsy is given in Table 16.4. The most commonly used drugs in the UK are carbamazepine, valproate and phenytoin, but worldwide, because of its cheapness, phenobarbitone is the most used antiepileptic.

Drug treatment of epilepsy

Not everybody who has a fit requires drug treatment. If a patient has had a single generalized fit with no demonstrable underlying pathology they have approximately a 50% chance of going on to get further fits. Most neurologists do not give drug treatment for first fits, unless there is underlying structural brain abnormality. If fits are very infrequent or very minor patients may elect not to take drug therapy. Alcoholics are notoriously non-compliant with medication. Drug treatment may merely add medication withdrawal to ethanol withdrawal as precipitants of seizures.

Surgical treatment of epilepsy

For that minority of patients with poorly controlled focal epilepsy surgery is an important consideration. The most performed and effective operation is temporal lobectomy. In well selected patients a 75% success rate is achievable, success being defined as cessation or marked reduction in the number of seizures. Patients who do well are those with a history of early childhood convulsions and MR abnorm-

Name Generic: **Phenytoin**   Proprietary: Epanutin
Types of epilepsy: focal or 1° & 2° tonic-clonic
Usual dose: 100 mg TID   *Levels*: 60–80 Tmol/l
   $T_{\frac{1}{2}}$: 24 hr
Toxic side effects: ataxia, nystagmus, blurred vision
Idiosyncratic side effects: coarse facial features, acne, hir-
   sutism, lupus, erythema multiforme, gingival hypertro-
   phy, megaloblastic anaemia, hepatitis
Teratogenicity: fetal hydantoin syndrome, cardiac, hair lip,
   cleft palate

Name Generic: **Valproate**   Proprietary: Epilim
Types of epilepsy: absence, focal, 1° & 2° tonic-clonic,
   myoclonic
Usual dose: 1–3 g/day   *Levels*: not useful $T_{\frac{1}{2}}$: 4–6 hr
Toxic side effects: tremor
Idiosyncratic side effects: hair loss, weight gain, hepatitis
Teratogenicity: 1% neural tube defect

Name Generic: **Carbamazepine**   Proprietary: Tegretol
Types of epilepsy: focal, 1° & 2° tonic-clonic
Usual dose: 400 mg TID   *Levels*: <50 Tmol/l, 4–12 mg/l
   $T_{\frac{1}{2}}$: 6–8 hr
Toxic side effects: drowsiness, diplopia, status epilepticus
Idiosyncratic side effects: rash, leucopenia, SIADH
Teratogenicity: cardiac, MR, neural tube

Name Generic: **Phenobarbitone**   Proprietary: none
Types of epilepsy: all except absence
Usual dose: 60–180 mg at night
   Levels: 60–180 µmol/l $T_{\frac{1}{2}}$: 100 hr
Toxic side effects: drowsiness, intellectual impairment,
   ataxia
Idiosyncratic side effects: rash, megaloblastic anaemia,
   hyperactivity (children)
Teratogenicity: fetal hydantoin syndrome

Name Generic: **Clonazepam**   Proprietary: Rivotril
Types of epilepsy: all forms, especially myoclonic
Usual dose: 4–8 mg/day   *Levels*: N/A $T_{\frac{1}{2}}$: long
Toxic side effects: drowsiness
Idiosyncratic side effects: abnormal LFTs
Teratogenicity: NK

Name Generic: **Vigabatrin**   Proprietary: Sabril
Types of epilepsy: focal and generalized tonic-clonic
Usual dose: 1 g b.d.   *Levels*: not done $T_{\frac{1}{2}}$: 4–5 hr
Toxic side effects: drowsiness and dizziness
Idiosyncratic side effects: psychosis
Teratogenicity: NK

Name Generic: **Lamotrigine**   Proprietary: Lamictal
Types of epilepsy: focal with secondary generalization
Usual dose: 200 mg b.d. (half dose if on valproate)
   Levels: not done $T_{\frac{1}{2}}$: 29 hr
Toxic side effects: ataxia, drowsiness
Idiosyncratic side effects: rash, exacerbation of epilepsy
Teratogenicity: NK

Name Generic: **Gabapentin**   Proprietary: Neurontin
Types of epilepsy: focal with secondary generalization

Usual dose: 400 mg t.d.s.   *Levels*: not done $T_{\frac{1}{2}}$: 5–7 hr
Toxic side effects: somnolence, ataxia
Idiosyncratic side effects: convulsions
Teratogenicity: NK

Name Generic: **Topiramate**   Proprietary: Topamax
Types of epilepsy: focal with secondary generalization
Usual dose: 100–300 mg b.d.   *Levels*: not done
Toxic side effects: drowsiness, ataxia
Idiosyncratic side effects: weight loss
Teratogenicity: yes in animals

Name Generic: **Ethosuximide**   Proprietary: Zarontin
Types of epilepsy: absence
Usual dose: 1–2 g/day   *Levels*: 300–700 µmol/l
Toxic side effects: drowsiness, ataxia
Idiosyncratic side effects: GI upset, rash, psychotic states
Teratogenicity: NK

Table 16.4 Antiepileptic drugs

alities supportive of a diagnosis of Ammond's horn sclerosis. Electrophysiological recordings are performed to help determine which temporal lobe is the source of the seizures, often involving sphenoidal electrodes. In addition, it has to be determined that the remaining temporal lobe is sufficient to maintain adequate memory. This is done by assessing the memory capability of each temporal lobe by putting the other one to sleep with amylobarbitone (Wada test).

Advice given to patients

Those few minutes during a consultation when a patient is told their diagnosis of epilepsy are some of the most important minutes in that person's life. How the news is given, the physician's attitude to epilepsy and the information given are crucial in how the patient will cope with their disease. Many patients are in shock and may not take in all the information given at that time. Subsequent appointments, nurse run clinics and written information are often very valuable. There are four general areas that need covering, general care, avoidance of hazardous situations, medication and driving (Tables 16.5–16.7).

Case history

Angela Cobridge is a 19-year-old woman who had been well until 2 years of age. At that time she developed a viral infection associated with a high fever and went into a prolonged seizure lasting just under 12 hours. During the next couple of days she had a weakness of the left side. She made an apparently full recovery until she was 8 years of age when she started having 'spells'. These would consist of her stopping whatever she was doing, becoming unresponsive and fiddling with her hands. Afterwards she would be dazed for a few seconds. Often she would feel tired after an attack. Initially she only had attacks once every month and they seemed to be responding to carbamazepine. By the time she was 15 she was getting daily attacks and was taking carbamazepine and valproate. Her school work was suffering. Her father had left the marital home and her mother was taking a greater and greater protective role in Angela's life. By the time she was 19 she had been tried on phenytoin, lamotrigine, gabapentin and vigabatrin; all with either unacceptable side effects or minimal effect on her epilepsy. Repeated EEGs had demonstrated epileptiform activity primarily arising from the right temporal lobe. An MR scan with quantitative assessment of the hippocampi had demonstrated right hippocampal atrophy. She had been started on the evaluation programme for consideration of temporal lobe surgery, but had found the process too psychologically stressful. Currently she is on carbamazepine 200 mg three times a day and 15 mg of phenobarbitone a day. The latter is being gradually increased. She is getting one to five attacks a day and is constantly in the company of her mother. She has never been employed and never goes out. She is a well presented, pleasant young woman whose life is devastated by her poorly controlled partial complex seizures which arise from Ammon's horn sclerosis.

Distance patient from potential hazards
Recovery position
Nothing in the mouth
Prolonged fit (>5–10 min) call an ambulance

Table 16.5 General care of someone having a generalized seizure

Work – machinery
Recreation – swimming (always accompanied)
Home – baths and bathroom doors
Precipitants – alcohol (OK in moderation)
              fatigue
              flashing lights (in the photosensitive)

Table 16.6 Avoidance of hazardous situations

A single seizure or unexplained loss of consciousness usually results in the loss of the driving licence for 1 year.
More than one seizure results in loss of licence until the patient has been fit free for 1 year.
If a patient has had only nocturnal seizures for 3 years then he/she can apply for a licence.
Any fits over the age of 5 years of age disqualify the patient from holding an HGV/PSV licence until they have been fit free and off medication for 10 years.
The law treats simple focal seizures (auras) the same as generalized.
The physician's role is to inform the patient and it is then the patient's responsibility to inform the driving licence authorities.

Table 16.7 Driving and epilepsy in the UK

The general care advice is primarily for relatives or friends. Most people who witness a generalized seizure for the first time think their loved one is going to die. A good starting point is to recognize how frightened they have been. A discussion of proposed medication should be focused on the patient's attitudes to taking medication, the importance of compliance, common side effects and rare severe side effects. Often drug regimens are complex and have to be written out for the patient as they will not remember them. Great confusion arises from the existence of proprietary and generic names. All advice has to be tempered with a sense of realism. The aim in treating epileptics is for the patient to live a normal life. Prescriptive advice to give up their job can be very destructive. It is better the patient is made aware of the level of risk they run and make their own mind up about what is and is not acceptable.

Driving is the major difficulty. Most patients do not realize that if they continue to drive and have not informed their insurance company they are not likely to be covered if a crash occurs and are personally liable. Again, an impartial presentation of the legal realities and allowing the patient to come to their own decision is usually the most effective method. However, one is legally obliged to break medical confidentiality and inform the authorities if one knows an epileptic is continuing to drive. Many physicians consider medical ethics take precedence over the law of the land.

Prescribing for females of child-bearing age

One must presume that all women from puberty to the menopause (unless sterilized) are in danger of becoming pregnant. So counselling and prescribing of antiepileptic drugs (AEDs) should take this reality into account. A large proportion of pregnancies are not planned and by the time the patient realizes she is pregnant it is half way through the first trimester and changes in antiepileptic regimens are too late to avoid teratogenicity. The risk is small, but real. Approximately 3% of babies born to normal mothers have some imperfection, 1% will be severe. Taking AEDs and having epilepsy approximately doubles the risk. Having epilepsy itself is a risk factor. Taking valproate in pregnancy produces a 1% risk of spina bifida. The safest drug is thought to be carbamazepine, but the evidence is not good. In principle, drug regimens should be reconsidered prior to conception. The question needs to be raised as to whether an AED is necessary at all. If an AED is needed then monotherapy with the lowest effective dose is the safest way to proceed. Folate supplementation should start prior to conception. Neural tube defects in those on valproate can be screened for though many women find the idea of a therapeutic termination difficult to cope with. In general, counselling should be reassuring and stress that it is very unlikely that your patient's baby will be anything other than perfect.

MCQs for Chapter 16

The MCQs are either true T or false F. The answers are given in Appendix 3. Negatively mark your answers; a point for a correct answer, deduct a point for an incorrect response. If you score 24 or more you pass.

1. **Key characteristics of epilepsy are:**
   A It is paroxysmal.
   B It is recurrent.
   C It is associated with loss of consciousness.
   D It is always associated with abnormalities on the surface EEG.

2. **The classification of epilepsy:**
   A Auras are frequently experienced in primary generalized epilepsy.
   B *Jamais vu* may be experienced in temporal lobe epilepsy.
   C Complex partial seizures involve alteration in the level of consciousness.
   D Myoclonic epilepsy is usually partial.

3. **Diagnosis:**
   A The diagnosis of epilepsy is clinical.
   B A sore tongue suggests a generalized seizure.
   C Flashing lights can precipitate a fit.
   D Headache is rarely seen in generalized epilepsy.

4.
   A Patients with focal epilepsy are more likely to have a relevant family history than those with primary generalized epilepsy.
   B Prolonged seizures in childhood are associated with temporal lobe epilepsy.
   C In older patients brain tumours rarely present with seizures.
   D MRI should not be used in children because of the radiation.

5. **Non-epileptic seizure disorder (NESD):**
   A NESD can be diagnosed with confidence on history alone.
   B 37% of patients with NESD have concurrent epilepsy.

C Confronting the patient with the diagnosis is often therapeutic.
D Urinary incontinence is common in NESD.

6. **Drug treatment:**
   A Is usually initiated after the first fit.
   B Alcoholics with epilepsy usually respond well to phenytoin.
   C Over 70% of patients are well controlled with standard drugs.
   D Carbamazepine and valproate are first line antiepileptic drugs.

7. **Side effects:**
   A Carbamazepine can cause leucopenia.
   B Valproate can cause hepatitis.
   C Phenytoin is suitable for adolescent females.
   D Vigabatrin can cause the fetal hydantoin syndrome.

8. **Advice for epileptics:**
   A Patients should be accompanied when swimming.
   B Alcohol is absolutely contraindicated.
   C Nothing should be put in the mouth during a fit.
   D Isolated short fits do not require hospitalization.

9. **Driving and epilepsy:**
   A Epileptics who are fit free for a year can apply for a driving licence.
   B Patients who have only nocturnal fits for 3 years can apply for a licence.
   C Patients having simple focal fits can drive.
   D It is the doctor's responsibility to inform the authorities.

10. **Prescribing for females of child-bearing age:**
    A The safest AED in pregnancy is thought to be phenytoin.
    B Valproate is associated with a 1% risk of spina bifida.
    C Folate supplements should be started at the end of the first trimester.
    D Monotherapy is important in reducing the risk of teratogenicity.

17. Central demyelination

Objectives

In this chapter we shall discuss the most common cause of disability in young adults after trauma: multiple sclerosis. Specific areas covered are:

- Multiple sclerosis   Epidemiology
                        Presentation
                        Examination
                        Investigations
                        Prognosis
                        Breaking bad news
- Treatment of MS
- Acute disseminated encephalomyelitis
- Optic neuritis

Basic science – the immune system

As in the peripheral nervous system, either the nerves or the myelin sheaths that surround them can be under pathological attack in the central nervous system. Damage to the myelin sheaths is called demyelination.

Multiple sclerosis

The commonest form of central demyelination is multiple sclerosis. It is a disease of unknown aetiology, but immunologically mediated, characterized pathologically by widespread occurrence in the central nervous system of patches of demyelination followed by gliosis. Clinically, dissemination of lesions in time and space are the characteristics of the condition. This common and disabling disorder is greatly feared by the general public. Its initial symptoms and signs can be quite subtle and there must be few neurologists who have not con-

sidered the possibility that they themselves are suffering from MS at some stage in their career.

Epidemiology

MS is common, about 1/800 Northern Europeans have the disorder. It has an interesting distribution in that it is more common in temperate regions than in the tropics (Table 17.1). There are two main theories to account for this observation. The first is that exposure to viral illnesses in childhood predisposes to developing MS later in life. There is some evidence that you take the risk of where you grew up with you if you emigrate. The other theory is that the observed differences are due to genes carried in Northern European stock and patterns of emigration account for the variation in distribution. Neither theory accounts for all the facts and one is reminded

Case history

Zoe Tunstall is a 23-year-old inspector for the government who visits farms to check on compliance with health and safety legislation. She presented to me with a 10-day history of pain behind the left eye which was worse on moving the eye, followed 2 days later by the reduction in vision in that eye to the point she could only just discern shapes. By the time I saw her her vision was beginning to improve in that she could see more detail, but colour perception in that eye was very poor. She had been feeling tired for the last 3 months and had fallen off her horse on three occasions that season. She was a keen point to point rider and the falls were most unusual. Two years previously she had had a numb foot, but had been re-assured by her GP that it was a 'trapped nerve' and would resolve spontaneously, which it did.

On examination she had a reduced visual acuity in the left eye down to 6/36 and poor red perception. There was a hint of nystagmus on left lateral gaze, but it was not sustained. Tone was minimally increased in the right leg.

As her eye was improving she received no specific treatment. An MR scan of the head demonstrated three areas of increased signal on T2 in the periventricular white matter suggestive of demyelination. Routine blood tests and a vasculitis screen were negative.

Six months later she returned to me with a 5-day history of numbness in the legs spreading up to her lower abdomen, with weakness in the legs to the point she could only just walk, and had urgency of micturition. In the intervening 6 months she had had a lot of 'pins and needles' in the hands. Her latest episode confirmed the diagnosis of MS which she had been told was a possibility when she had had her optic neuritis. She underwent a 3-day course of 1 g methylprednisolone intravenously daily and within a month had made a near full recovery from her transverse myelitis. She has given up riding point to point and because of the fatigue does her job but has no energy for recreational activities.

10/100 000 in New Orleans
41/100 000 in Boston
129/100 000 in Northern Canada

Table 17.1 Variation of incidence of MS within North America

siblings of someone with MS, a 1/20 chance. Monozygotic twins have a 30% concordance, but put the other way around, even with identical genetic material, there is a 70% chance of not developing MS; much of the variance is not genetic in origin. There are associations with DRB1 and DQB1 of the class II MHC. These associations are hypothesized to relate to antigen presentation and recognition between lymphocyte subpopulations.

Presentation

Patients present with a single episode of demyelination which usually resolves over a few weeks (Table 17.2). If a careful history is obtained there may have been previous episodes which on occasion are sufficiently clear cut to allow a clinical diagnosis to be made. Direct questions should ask about diplopia, visual loss, weakness and numbness in the limbs. A single clinical attack of MS does not allow the diagnosis to be made. A colleague of mine (Giles Elrington) has coined the term monosclerosis to describe this situation.

Examination

A detailed neurological examination may reveal abnormalities that suggest previous episodes of demyelination that have been forgotten about or were subclinical. Pale optic discs and loss of colour vision are signs of previous optic neuritis. Nystagmus, diplopia

18% Weakness in both lower limbs
14% Weakness in one lower limb
16% Blindness in one eye
11% Numbness or paraesthesiae

Table 17.2 The initial attack in MS

of those sterile nature versus nurture arguments that used to rage over intelligence. The offspring of someone with MS have a 1/50 chance of developing the disease. The or an internuclear ophthalmoplegia (see Chapter 10) suggest previous brain-stem demyelination. Bilateral long track signs such as hyper-reflexia and Babinski's sign imply a previous myelopathy and dystaxia of the limbs or gait and may suggest cerebellar involvement.

Investigations

There are a number of investigations available to help confirm the diagnosis (Table 17.3). Sometimes the history is so classical that investigation is hardly necessary; however, once a diagnosis of MS has been made it is difficult to unmake it. A foramen magnum lesion, brain stem and spinal arteriovenous malformation, familial spastic paraplegia, adult onset leucodystrophy, lupus, sarcoid and Behçet's can all mimic MS.

MRI of the brain shows abnormalities in 98% of patients with clinically definite MS. However, the investigation is not specific and similar white matter abnormalities can be seen due to ischaemia as with advancing age or cerebral vasculitis. MRI is often used as a screening tool in patients presenting with symptoms possibly suggestive of MS. Under these circumstances the sensitivity of the test is likely to be far lower than the 98% in established disease. In patients with a single clinical episode (monosclerosis) the presence of abnormalities on MRI makes it likely they will develop clinical MS within the next 5 years, while an absence of lesions makes it unlikely they will develop MS in the medium term. Gadolinium is used to demonstrate

breakdown of the blood–brain barrier, which is the first event in the development of an MS plaque. It increases the number of abnormalities seen, but significantly adds to the cost of the investigation. MRI of the cord is usually performed to exclude structural lesions, but plaques can also be demonstrated.

Evoked potentials are useful in establishing evidence of subclinical disease in pathways not known to be affected, so contributing to the clinical criteria of disease disseminated in time and space (for methodology see Chapter 10). They are also useful in patients in whom the organic basis of the disorder is in doubt. MRI of the spine is variable in its sensitivity in picking up plaques and in patients with purely cord disease the MRI of the head may be normal. Lower limb sensory evoked potentials will then demonstrate delay.

The cerebrospinal fluid may show a mild lymphocytic pleocytosis (up to 50 cells/mm^3) and moderately raised protein, particularly during exacerbations. Eighty-five per cent of patients with MS will demonstrate an increase in intrathecal immunoglobulin synthesis or oligoclonal bands. However, these changes are not specific and other disorders that give rise to abnormalities on MRI also produce oligoclonal bands.

Prognosis

There are four main prognostic groups which can only be differentiated with certainty in retrospect. They are relapsing and remitting with accumulating disability (60%), progressive from onset, with or without superimposed relapses (10%), malignant (10%) and benign (10%). Malignant means rapid progression to severe disability over a few weeks. Benign involves a few relapses, but no or little disability over many years. Patients who are younger, female and present with purely sensory symptoms have a more favourable prognosis than older male patients with progressive motor problems. The overall prognosis is that 20% die of their disease and its complications, 60% are disabled, 20% remain not disabled. There may be a further 20% who have very

MRI ± gadolinium
  Brain
  Spinal cord
Evoked potentials
  VEP
  SEP
  BAEP
CSF
  Oligoclonal bands
  IgG synthetic rate

Table 17.3 Tests used in multiple sclerosis

mild disease who have not come to medical attention. All these figures are approximate and depend on the duration of follow up. The longer patient cohorts are followed up the worse the prognosis appears, but with the advent of MRI milder cases are being diagnosed which may shift the overall prognosis in a more favourable direction.

Breaking bad news

Telling someone they have multiple sclerosis is one of the most important moments in their life. There are frequent complaints that this delicate job is done in a ham-fisted insensitive fashion. Some of these complaints may be deflected anger, but too many are justified. The principles of giving bad news are given in Table 17.4. The structural aspects of the setting are important. An open medical ward is probably the worst possible place to deliver bad news. Ideally there should be a quiet, pleasantly furnished room where privacy can be assured. The seating should all be at the same level. There needs to be enough time set aside for this task, which may not be long, but should not be pressured. The interview itself should start by making sure everyone knows who everyone else is. The topic to be discussed should be introduced. Often a résumé of the course of events that have led up to the present is a sensible way to proceed. The bad news should be given in clear unambiguous language and then the receiver should be given an opportunity to express themselves and ask questions. Large amounts of factual information given at this time will not be remembered. Some discussion of the way forward is appropriate and then a summary at the end of the interview will bring it to a close. Patients and relatives need to feel they have access when further questions arise and there should be communication with the rest of the team involved in the patient's care both inside and outside the hospital. Ideally there should be continuity of care with the patient being seen by people he or she already knows and trusts.

Structural aspects
Undisturbed privacy
Time
Appropriate seating and room
The interview
Introduction
Information clear and non-technical: but limit information load initially
Allow patient/relative to express self
Open questions
Explicit permission to express emotion
Silence, eye contact and non-verbal communication
What now
Summarize
Follow up
Access
Team work – communication
Continuity of care

Table 17.4 The principles of giving bad news

Treatment of MS

It is incorrect to say there is no treatment for multiple sclerosis, but there is no cure (Table 17.5). Most acute episodes are self-limiting and require no intervention other than reassurance. Where the episode is disabling (in the patient's eyes) then steroids are worth considering. For major disabling episodes many neurologists would use high dose intravenous methylprednisolone (500 mg for 5 days or 1 g for 3 days). These short courses are relatively free of side effects, but patients need to be warned of the risks of mood changes, heightening of facial colour, hypertension, transient diabetes and although it is rare, because it is permanent, avascular necrosis of the hip. The response to steroids takes between 3 days and 3 weeks. It is thought not to have any effect on long-term prognosis. Until recently disease altering treatments were fairly limited. Immunosuppression with azathioprine reduced relapse rate, but the effect was modest and the potential side effects worrisome.

Beta-interferon looks like a major advance in the treatment of MS. It reduces the frequency of lesions appearing on MRI and clinical disability. There are two forms of β-interferon, 1A and 1B. Both can produce neutralizing antibodies to β-interferon. There

Basic science – the immune system

The immune system is complex and at least some of the complexity is a result of our ignorance and the opaqueness of the nomenclature. There are important general concepts that can be lost in the detail so I shall endeavour to keep things simple.

There are two main divisions in the immune response, the humoral, which is dependent on antibody secretion by B-lymphocytes and their plasma cell progeny and the cell-mediated response which is dependent on T-lymphocytes. In general, B cells and antibodies kill bacteria while cytotoxic T cells kill viruses.

Antibodies

IgG is composed of two light chains and two heavy chains. The N-terminal domains of both light and heavy chains are very variable and contain the antigen binding site. The constant domain of the heavy chains determines the subtype of antibody (IgG, A, D, M or E).

IgG is the major immunoglobulin in the secondary immune response. It is the only Ig to cross the placenta.

IgA is the primary Ig secreted onto mucous membranes and in tears and saliva. It helps protect the respiratory and gastrointestinal tracts against infection.

IgM is made of five subunits and is the principal immunoglobulin in the primary response.

IgD is thought to be related to B-cell activity.

IgE causes mast cells to degranulate and is associated with immediate hypersensitivity reactions.

Lymphocytes

B-cells recognize antigen with surface receptors, but require further stimuli from T helper cells in order to produce antibody. T cells recognize antigen on cell surfaces.

T cells are subdivided into cytotoxic (which can lyse cells, e.g. a virus infected cell) and T-helper cells which activate B cells and other lymphocytes.

Natural killer cells are large granular lymphocytes which are neither T nor B and are activated by interferon.

Histocompatibility (HLA) molecules

On the presenting cell the antigen has to be presented by the histocompatibility (HLA) molecules. HLA antigens are encoded in the major histocompatibility complex (MHC) on the short arm of chromosome 6.

Class I HLA are present on most cells and display abnormal antigens if they are present, for example if the cell is infected with a virus. Some cells lack HLA class I, such as tumour cells, and some have only very low levels, like hepatocytes, muscle and nerve cells. Expression by HLA I is increased by interferon γ.

Class II HLA is expressed on the surface of B lymphocytes, monocytes, activated T cells and some epithelial cells. Class II HLA present foreign-derived antigen to T-helper cells. T cells need to be activated in order to interact with antigen presenting cells. This is facilitated by adhesion molecules and also B7 which binds to T-helper cell glycoprotein CD28. This signals to naïve T cells to initiate a response.

T-helper cells carry the CD4 on their surface which interacts with antigen presented by the HLA class II on a presenting cell. There may be two classes of T-helper cells, Th_1 and Th_2. Th_1 secrete IL-2, interferon γ, and they mediate cellular immunity. Th_2 secrete IL-4, -5, and -10 which are involved in humoral immunity. Cytotoxic lymphocytes release lymphokines, interferon and tumour necrosis factor.

Cytotoxic T cells carry the CD8 which is involved in the recognition of HLA class II presented antigen receptor.

Cytokines

Cytokines are small polypeptides which include IL-1-12, IF-γ and TNF. They are secreted by lymphocytes and have a number of functions including activation of lymphocytes, proliferation and chemotaxis.

Complement

Complement is a cascade of enzymes that ends in cell lysis and produces lymphocyte chemotaxis and immobilization of lymphocytes along the way. It is activated by antigen-antibody complexes or some antigens such as endotoxin or lipopolysaccharide.

is some evidence that efficacy can be lost in the presence of these antibodies. It is thought that 1B is more likely to produce antibodies than 1A. 1A has been demonstrated to slow the development of disability. The cost of these drugs has led to a major delay in their availability to patients in the UK. Other disease altering drugs are at various stages of development including copolymer 1. In future there will be a variety of agents available to the patient and clinician that have an effect on disease progression.

Many patients develop a spastic paraparesis. Where spasticity and spasms are the major problems antispasmodics such as baclofen can be useful. They tend to increase weakness so a balance has to be struck between their advantages and disadvantages. Urgency and urinary incontinence are common symptoms in spinal MS. The anticholinergic drugs can be helpful. Later intermittent self-catheterization can provide an answer, but it relies on having enough dexterity in the hands and truncal control, or a willing partner in order to do it. Permanent indwelling catheters are a solution, but frequently become infected. Sepsis often results in a worsening of the symptoms of MS as an elevated temperature makes saltatory transmission less effective. Patients with MS are prone to hypostatic and aspiration pneumonia, urinary tract infection and infection in decubiti ulcers.

Physiotherapy and occupational therapy are important aspects of maintaining function in patients with MS. There are a few patients in whom tremor is the most disabling symptom. Ventrolateral thalotomy has been used successfully in a small number of patients.

Acute disseminated encephalomyelitis (ADEM)

ADEM is the Guillain–Barré of the CNS. It is a single phase illness that occurs a few days to 3 weeks after a minor (usually upper respiratory tract) infection. Multiple areas of the central nervous system are damaged simultaneously. There is disagreement as to over what

Acute episodes
Oral steroids
Intravenous high dose steroids
ACTH
Disease altering
β-Interferon 1A and 1B
Immunosuppression – azathioprine
Spasm/increased tone
Baclofen
Dantrolene
Diazepam
Urinary incontinence
Anticholinergics
Intermittent self-catheterization
Permanent indwelling catheter
Immobility
Physiotherapy and physical aids
Sepsis
Lung
Urinary tract
Decubitii
Tremor
Ventrolateral thalotomy

Table 17.5 Treatments for multiple sclerosis

period lesions are allowed to evolve, but the more temporally restricted the less likely ADEM will turn out to be its main differential, MS. There is a hyperacute form of ADEM with pyrexia, generalized encephalopathy, fever, a polymorph pleocytosis in the CSF and an appreciable mortality. The more usual ADEM often has a mixed lymphocyte and polymorph pleocytosis in the CSF. There is a rationale for using high doses of intravenous steroids in the treatment of this condition. Oligoclonal bands are often positive during the attack, but subsequently become negative. In MS they continue to be positive. The initial MRI cannot differentiate ADEM from MS; however, if an MRI is repeated a couple of months after the initial assault and there are fresh gadolinium-enhancing lesions seen then the final diagnosis is likely to be MS. Similar postviral monophasic episodes of CNS damage can be seen following rubella, measles, pertussis, scarlet fever and vaccination. There is a chronic subacute form with a poor prognosis following measles called subacute sclerosing panencephalitis. A similar condition can be seen after rubella.

Optic neuritis

Optic neuritis may be an isolated event or be the harbinger of multiple sclerosis. It usually starts with pain on moving the eye followed by visual loss over hours or days to a nadir which may be mild fuzziness of vision to complete blindness. Colour vision may be particularly affected. Recovery takes weeks. Ninety per cent of patients consider they have made a full recovery, buy careful testing reveals deficits in 50%. There is some data to suggest that high dose intravenous steroids improve the outcome, however in practice most unilateral cases run their natural course. The differential diagnosis is with ischaemic optic neuropathy, optic nerve sarcoidosis, and Leber's hereditary optic neuropathy. The risk of progression to MS is paradoxically lower if both eyes are affected. In a series of patients presenting with apparent optic neuritis 20% had MS at presentation, 5% had a conversion disorder, 15% had another disorder. Of the remaining patients 60% had developed clinical MS within $3\frac{1}{2}$ years.

MCQs for Chapter 17

The MCQs are either true T or false F. The answers are given in Appendix 3. Negatively mark your answers; a point for a correct answer, deduct a point for an incorrect response. If you score 24 or more you pass.

1. Multiple sclerosis:
   A Is immunologically mediated.
   B Has an incidence in Northern Europe of 1/100.
   C Is common in the tropics.
   D Monozygotic twins have a 30% concordance.

2. Multiple sclerosis:
   A A single clinical attack allows the diagnosis to be made.
   B Internuclear ophthalmoplegia is very suggestive of MS.
   C Cerebellar signs are rare.
   D A pale disc may be a sign of previous optic neuritis.

3. Investigating MS:
   A MRI of the brain is highly specific for MS.
   B Gadolinium enhancement demonstrates breakdown of the blood–brain barrier.
   C Evoked potentials can demonstrate subclinical disease.
   D Oligoclonal bands are specific for MS.

4. The prognosis in MS:
   A About 10% of patients with MS have benign disease.
   B The majority of patients have relapsing remitting disease.
   C Motor symptoms are a good prognostic sign.
   D Older patients have a worse prognosis.

5. Breaking bad news:
   A An open medical ward is a good place to tell someone they have MS.

   B The doctor should be seated higher than the patient.
   C Patients need large amounts of information when given bad news.
   D Continuity of care is important in giving bad news.

6. The side effects of steroids include:
   A Diabetes.
   B Hypertension.
   C Avascular necrosis of the hip.
   D Discoloured urine.

7. The treatment of MS:
   A Methylprednisolone maintains remission.
   B Beta-interferon reduces relapse rate.
   C Baclofen increases muscle strength.
   D Anticholinergics can be used for urgency.

8. Sepsis in MS:
   A Elevated temperature improves saltatory transmission.
   B MS sufferers are prone to meningitis.
   C Aspiration pneumonia is a complication of MS.
   D Urinary tract infection is common in longterm MS sufferers.

9. Acute disseminated encephalomyelitis:
   A Has multiple phases.
   B Only a single area of the CNS is usually affected.
   C May be accompanied by a fever.
   D Steroids are used acutely.

10. Optic neuritis:
   A Is often associated with discomfort.
   B Colour vision may be partially affected.
   C MS rarely develops following unilateral optic neuritis.
   D Optic neuritis rarely recovers completely.

18. Movement disorders

Objectives

In this chapter you will become acquainted with the clinical features and management of:

- Parkinsonism
- Parkinson's disease
- Other akinetic rigid syndromes
- Other movement disorders   Huntington's disease
  Friedreich's ataxia
  Dystonia
  Idiopathic torsion dystonia
  Gilles de la Tourette syndrome
  Tremor
  Neuroleptic-induced movement
    disorders

Basic science – free radicals and trinucleotide repeats

The movement disorders are a group of afflictions where the impression the patient makes on the observer is diagnostic. As pattern recognition is the key to their diagnosis only exposure to these conditions will allow the clinician to develop an awareness of the range of presentations. This also means that there can be disagreement between experts as into which diagnostic category a patient may fall.

Parkinsonism

There are a number of disorders that have akinesia (slow movements) and rigidity as central features. The most common is Parkinson's disease. Others include postencephalitic Parkinsonism, multisystem atrophy (Shy–

Drager) and progressive supranuclear palsy (Steele–Richardson–Olszewski) (Table 18.1).

Parkinson's disease (PD)

James Parkinson, a general practitioner in Shoreditch, London, described paralysis agitans in 1817. Parkinson's disease is an idiopathic disorder characterized by slowness of emotional and voluntary movement (bradykinesia), muscle rigidity and tremor.

Epidemiology

Parkinson's disease (PD) has an overall incidence of 1–2/1000, which makes it one of the most common neurological diseases. It is much more common in the over-50s age group. The

Parkinson's disease (idiopathic Parkinsonism)
Postencephalitic Parkinsonism – encephalitis lethargica
  1920s
Drug induced – dopamine antagonists
Atherosclerotic Parkinsonism
Toxins
  Manganese
  Carbon monoxide poisoning
  MPTP
Brain tumour
'Punch-drunk syndrome'
Degenerative diseases
  Corticostriatonigral degeneration
  Progressive supranuclear palsy
  Multisystem atrophy
  Parkinsonism – dementia complex of Guam

Table 18.1 The differential diagnosis of Parkinsonism

peak age of onset is between 55 and 70. There is a slight male preponderance.

Pathology

Pathologically at autopsy the substantia nigra can be seen to have lost pigmentation. There is degeneration of the nigrostriate pathway with loss of dopaminergic input into the striatum. Lewy bodies, acidophilic intracytoplasmic bodies surrounded by a paler zone, are found in the substantia nigra.

Clinical findings

The diagnosis of PD is usually made as the patient walks into the consulting room. The face is impassive, the posture slightly stooped and there is poor arm swing. The gait may be festinating with many small steps and the centre of gravity is moved anteriorly as if the patient is using the possibility of falling on his face as a means of propelling himself forward. The lack of facial expression means that the usual cues that moderate social interactions are absent, giving the impression that the patient is cold and unfeeling. Depression occurs in up to 90% of cases and dementia also develops in a proportion of patients as the disease progresses. The spouse of one of my patients kindly provided a description of her husband's condition which was diagnostic in itself (Fig. 18.1).

On examination the patient has increased tone in the limbs which is rigidity not spasticity. In spasticity the degree of resistance to movement varies with the speed of the movement. Often the clasp-knife phenomenon can be demonstrated where resistance is initially high then suddenly gives way. Resistance is usually higher when working against antigravity muscles. In rigidity the resistance is constant and not isolated to any particular muscle group. It is sometimes called 'lead pipe' rigidity as it is supposed to be akin to bending a lead pipe. The rigidity is reinforced when the opposite limb is in action. So the patient can be asked to wave their opposite arm up and down or open and close the opposite fist. In addition to rigidity a superimposed catch can be felt called cogwheeling. Some authors believe that this is due to a superimposed tremor on top of the rigidity, but I have never been impressed with this explanation. The signs are usually unilateral initially, but become bilateral after a few months. Rapid successive and alternating movements are slowed (bradykinesia) and deteriorating writing is characteristic. It tends to be small, getting smaller and undecipherable as the patient continues to write (Fig. 18.2). The tremor is classically a 'pill rolling movement', 4–6 Hz, and present at rest; however, an action tremor is not uncommon. Speech may be slurred, quiet and monotonous. Postural reflexes are often impaired. This can be tested by trying to push the patient over having first placed oneself in the path of their predicted trajectory. It would be unfortunate for a patient to fall during the examination. Patients with PD blink frequently and the glabellar tap is positive. Usually if you tap someone on their forehead they will rapidly stop blinking as the reflex becomes desensitized; however, patients with PD continue to blink.

Prognosis

While some patients can remain stable for up to 30 years most patients are significantly disabled within 10 years. Clues as to the

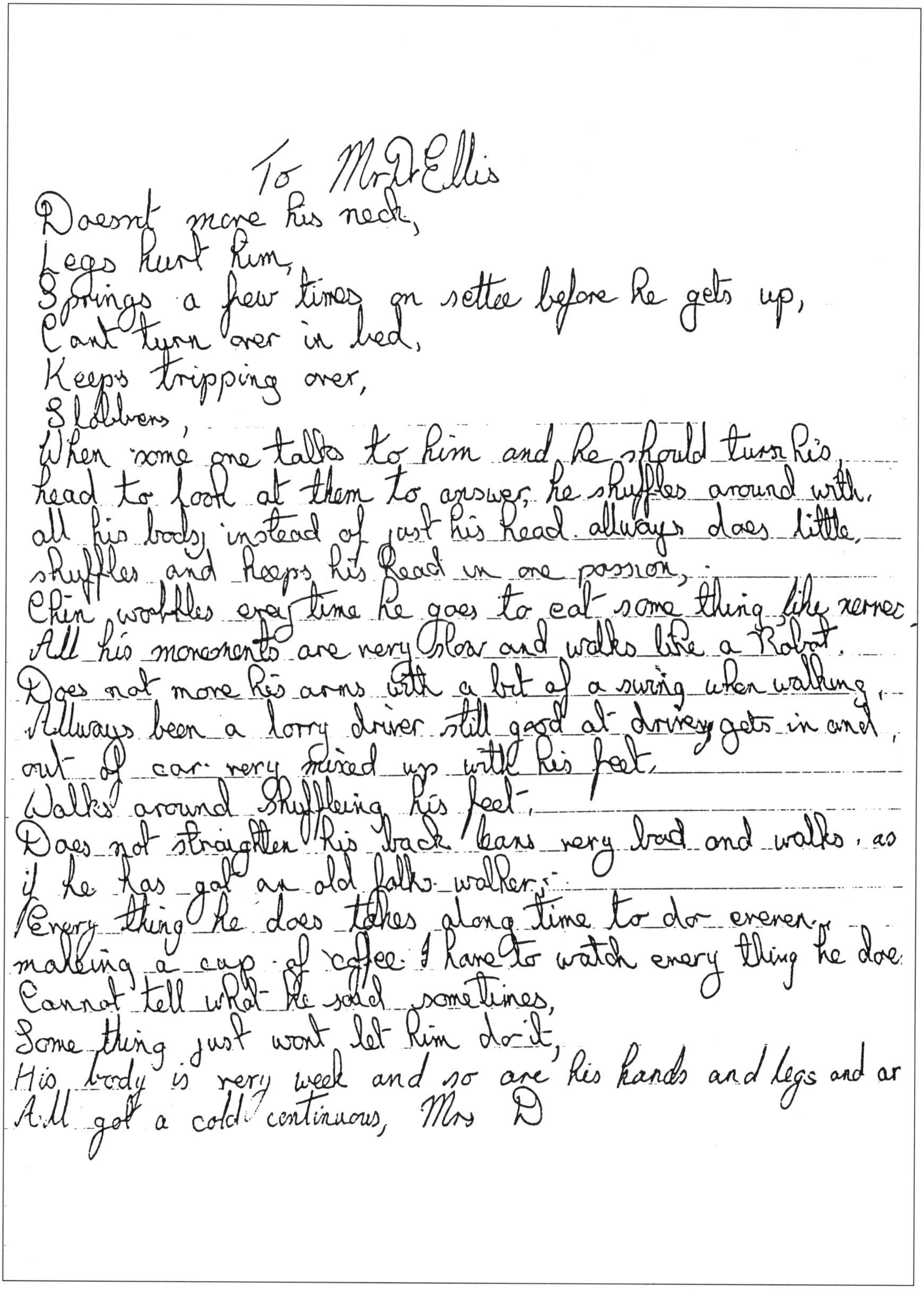

To Mr Dr Ellis

Doesnt move his neck,
Legs hurt him,
Springs a few times on settee before he gets up,
Cant turn over in bed,
Keeps tripping over,
Slobbers,
When some one talks to him and he should turn his
head to look at them to answer, he shuffles around with
all his body, instead of just his head. allways does little
shuffles and keeps his head in one passion,
Chin wobbles every time he goes to eat some thing like nerves,
All his movements are very slow and walks like a Robot.
Does not move his arms with a bit of a swing when walking,
Allways been a lorry driver still good at driving gets in and
out of car very mixed up with his feet,
Walks around shuffling his feet,
Does not straighten his back bans very bad and walks, as
if he has got an old folks walker,
Every thing he does takes along time to do evenen
making a cup of coffee I have to watch every thing he doe
Cannot tell what he said sometimes,
Some thing just wont let him do it,
His body is very week and so are his hands and legs and ar
All got a cold continuous, Mrs D

Fig. 18.1 Description of Parkinson's disease by patient's spouse.

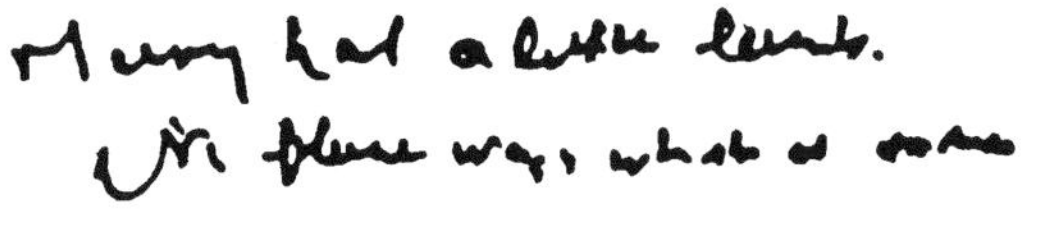

Fig. 18.2 Example of Parkinsonian writing.

prognosis are given by the patient's age (younger patients usually have a more protracted course) and the speed of development of the disease so far. Death is usually as a complication of immobility with orthostatic pneumonia as a leading cause. Many of the deaths occur at night and nocturnal sleep apnoea may play a role.

Treatment

Melvin Yahr (an American neurologist and expert on PD) describes Parkinson's disease as capricious. This has to be borne in mind when treating it. Changes in treatment regimens should only be made slowly as one day may not be the same as the next (Table 18.2).

The most effective treatment for PD is to give L-dopa which is converted in the brain by dopadecarboxylase to dopamine. In the rest of the body the conversion of L-dopa to dopamine would give rise to postural hypotension, nausea and vomiting so a dopadecarboxylase inhibitor, which cannot cross the blood–brain barrier, is given concurrently. These combination medications are available in the Sinemet and Madopar range of products. Only a committee could have arrived at the unwieldy generic names of co-careldopa and co-beneldopa, respectively. There are a variety of dosages and slow release versions available.

The major short-term side effects are still nausea and postural hypotension. In the longer term, particularly in the elderly, confusion and hallucinations are often the dose-limiting factors. There are concerns over the long-term effects of L-dopa, particularly the development of troublesome dyskinesias, and fluctuations in the effectiveness of the drugs as the disease advances. Some neurologists prefer to start patients either on an anticholinergic or a

Case history

Mrs Norton was a 53-year-old primary school teacher who had noticed a 'paralysis' in her left hand for 3 months. She thought she might have had a stroke and consulted her GP. Her GP asked for an urgent neurological outpatient appointment to exclude a space-occupying lesion. On taking a detailed history it emerged that Mrs Norton had found that she could not run as well as previously and this she attributed to her left foot. In addition, she had given up knitting as she found it difficult. Examination revealed a paucity of facial movement, which initially gave the impression that Mrs Norton was depressed. There was increased tone in the left arm with cogwheeling when the other hand was opened and closed. Strength and sensation were normal. Rapid successive movements were slowed on the left. All the deep tendon reflexes were present and her plantar responses were flexor. When she walked she did not swing her left arm. A diagnosis of Parkinson's disease was made and she was started on Sinemet Plus, one tablet twice a day, to increase to three times a day after 1 month. After some transitory nausea she settled well on her treatment and at review after 3 months said she felt better than she had for years. Her face was more expressive and her rigidity in the left hand had all but gone. She had started knitting again.

She was followed in the neurology clinic over the next 5 years with various adjustments to her anti-Parkinsonian regimen. She retired from teaching and developed stiffness and slowness of movements in the right hand. At the end of 7 years she was taking Sinemet CR (one tablet three times a day), Sinemet Plus (one tablet in the morning) and Pergolide (500 µg three times a day). She was able to walk reasonably well, but had had a fall. Her neurologist had noted peak dose dyskinesias, but these did not bother Mrs Norton as much as those observing her. She had had a couple of freezing episodes.

One would expect increasing difficulty over the next few years in balancing the anti-Parkinsonian effect of her medication against the side effects. Within the next 5 years or so Mrs Norton is likely to become severely disabled with her Parkinson's disease and will be prone to the illnesses that kill immobile patients such as chest infections.

L-Dopa/peripheral dopadecarboxylase inhibitor
Sinemet
Madopar
Anticholinergics
Benzhexol
Orphenadrine
Dopamine agonists
Bromocriptine
Pergolide
Apomorphine
β-MAOI inhibitor
Selegeline
Amantadine
Surgical
Ventrolateral thalotomy
Transplantation

Table 18.2 Treatments in Parkinson's disease

dopa agonist and save the L-dopa preparations for later.

The theory underlying the use of anticholinergics is that in the basal ganglia the cholinergic and dopaminergic systems are working in competition. By inhibiting the cholinergic system one can restore a balance. The anticholinergic drugs are supposed to be particularly effective against tremor, but of the three cardinal features of PD, tremor is often the most resistant to treatment. The anticholinergics cause constipation, retention of urine, dry mouth, they worsen glaucoma and have a particular propensity for worsening confusion.

The dopamine agonists are gaining in favour. They are used by some neurologists as the initial treatment and later in the disease they can have a role when the L-dopa preparations are less effective and fluctuations are a major problem. Confusion is unfortunately often a dose-limiting side effect.

There are theoretical reasons for believing that the β-MAOI inhibitor selegeline slows the progression of PD.* There is some methodologically flawed data to support this contention, however proof is lacking. Selegeline does have a mild anti-Parkinsonian effect and it prolongs and enhances the effects of the L-dopa preparations. In an open study an increased mortality was found in patients receiving selegeline, but their requirement for Sinemet stabilized rather than increased, year on year. This result has raised doubts over the safety of selegeline. My current initial regimen consists of one $\frac{1}{2}$ Sinemet CR twice a day and 10 mg of selegeline.

Amantadine promotes the synthesis and release of dopamine. Ventrolateral thalotomy is very rarely used for resistant tremor. Transplantation of fetal dopamine producing cells into the striatum of Parkinsonian patients is a promising if limited experimental therapy.

Other akinetic rigid syndromes

Multisystem atrophy (Shy–Drager syndrome)

Multisystem atrophy is an akinetic rigid syndrome with autonomic failure as a cardinal component, that may or may not have cerebellar features. Pathologically there is striatonigral degeneration, olivopontine atrophy and degeneration of the autonomic nervous system. The onset is usually in the fifth decade with autonomic symptoms such as impotence, incontinence and postural hypotension often predating the movement disorder. The patients are often unstable and fall frequently. There is little or no response to L-dopa. Sleep

---

* *The MPTP story*

In the 1980s the selective toxicity of MPTP for the substantia nigra was appreciated. Thanks to some pioneering experimental work on themselves, drug addicts, initially on the east coast of the United States and then on the west coast, became Parkinsonian after injecting novel drugs. The active agent was found to be MPTP and its metabolite MPP$^+$. This work was reproduced in monkeys who were protected from Parkinsonism if they were pretreated with selegeline. This has given rise to the theory for the genesis of Parkinson's disease that there is an environmental toxin which selectively damages the substantia nigra in genetically susceptible people. Following this line of thought it was hoped that neuroprotective agents could be developed to stop further degeneration. Selegeline was the first putative neuroprotective agent.

Basic science – free radicals

Free radicals have been considered potentially important in the development of many degenerative and inflammatory diseases including Parkinson's disease, atherosclerosis and rheumatoid arthritis. A free radical is any atom or molecule that contains one or more unpaired electrons. Usually the unpaired electron makes the molecule more reactive. The actions of free radicals are opposed in the body by antioxidants. Examples of these are vitamin C, vitamin E and beta-carotene. Antioxidants are also made in the body. They protect against oxygen toxicity. The harmful effect of oxygen can be seen in premature babies who are given 100% oxygen and develop retrolental fibroplasia. Oxygen toxicity is due to an excess formation of superoxide radical ($O_2^{\cdot -}$). Superoxide dismutase (SOD) enzymes remove this. Gamma radiation can split water into hydroxyl radicals $H^{\cdot}$ and $OH^{\cdot}$. These can attack proteins, lipids and DNA.

In Parkinson's disease there is increased free radical damage to DNA. A 40% drop in reduced glutathione (GSH) is found in PD. GSH is needed by glutathione peroxidase to remove H_2O_2.

apnoea occurs and the mean duration of the illness is only 5 years from diagnosis to death.

Progressive supranuclear palsy (PSP) (Steele–Richardson–Olszewski syndrome)

PSP is another akinetic rigid syndrome, but with eye movement abnormalities as a prominent feature. A supranuclear palsy is a disorder of eye movement that cannot be accounted for by a cranial nerve nuclei problem. The earliest problem in PSP is often with vertical gaze. Often the patients cannot voluntarily look upwards, but if the eyes are fixed on a target and the head is moved then more upward movement is obtained. As the disease progresses there is increasing axial rigidity, extension of the neck, intellectual impairment and ophthalmoplegia. PET and SPECT scanning demonstrate frontal hypometabolism. Again there is a poor response to L-dopa.

Other movement disorders

Huntington's disease (chorea)

Huntington's disease (chorea) is an autosomal dominant condition due to a CAG repeat on

Case history

Ian Smallheath was an electrician with the city council. He was brought to see a neurologist when he was 45 years old by a family friend. Ten years previously he had had a couple of episodes of depression which had been successfully treated by his GP. He had been a fully qualified electrical engineer, but 3 years previously had been down-graded to storesman. Six months prior to my seeing him he had been further down-graded and now only undertook simple menial tasks. A head injury at work had been the precipitant for him coming to medical attention. He lived on his own and his only close contact was a family friend. His father and uncle had died of Huntington's chorea. His sister lived in another town and did not keep in contact. On examination he appeared to be constantly on the move with small choreiform movements that give the impression of extreme anxiety. He made a couple of errors on the mini-mental test, but was only moderately impaired. A clinical diagnosis of Huntington's chorea was made and after counselling he had the blood test for the CAG repeat. On one chromosome there were 15 repeats, but on the other there were 43, clearly in the pathological range. He continued to have accidents at work and was finally retired on health grounds. He became bored and despondent living on his own with nothing to do. Community psychiatric nursing services were called in to support him. His cognitive abilities and co-ordination will decline over the next few years. It will become impossible to care for him in the community and he will require some form of institutional care. He will end up immobile and demented, finally succumbing to a pneumonia or sepsis from a urinary tract infection.

the short arm of chromosome 4 with an incidence in the UK of 1/14 000. In each successive generation the number of repeats can lengthen shortening the time to onset of the disease. The disorder manifests itself as choreiform movements, tics, and progressive dementia. Death occurs about 12 years after diagnosis. Episodes of depression can predate the more florid manifestations. There is a rigid akinetic variant that can occur in younger patients. The usual age of onset is 25–55, but since the gene has been detectable it has been found that a number of elderly patients with 'senile chorea' have an excessive number of CAG repeats. There is atrophy of the caudate nucleus which is demonstrable on CT later in the disease. GABA levels are low. The chorea can be suppressed with tetrabenazine (an amine depleting agent, which can precipitate depression), haloperidol or sulparide. Now the gene can be detected individuals in affected families can be screened. This requires skilled counselling before and after. Interestingly, individuals with a negative test can have trouble adjusting to a life without the threat of Huntington's.

Friedreich's ataxia

This is the most common early onset ataxia with a prevalence of 1–2/100 000. As an adult neurologist I rarely ever see a case. It is an autosomal recessive disorder consisting of degeneration of the posterior columns and spinocerebellar tracts in the spinal cord. It presents between 8 and 15 years of age with progressive limb and gait ataxia, absent deep tendon reflexes in the lower limbs and electrophysiological evidence of an axonal sensory neuropathy. Later, dysarthria, pyramidal weakness in the legs, loss of proprioception and vibration sense in the legs and extensor plantar responses develop. Optic atrophy occurs in about a quarter of cases.

Dystonia

The term dystonia refers to any abnormality of muscle tone, but it is usually used in a more restricted fashion. Aficionados of movement

---

Basic science – genetics: trinucleotide repeats

A number of genetic disorders are being attributed to trinucleotide repeats. These include Huntington's chorea and Friedreich's ataxia, fragile X syndrome and a number of rarer neurological illnesses.

Throughout the normal genome there are short repetitive sequences. In normal people there are between 11 and 30 repeats of the three bases, cytosine (C), adenine (A), and guanine (G) on the Huntington's gene (4p16.3). If there are excessive repeats then there is a high likelihood of developing Huntington's disease. Greater than 36 CAG repeats is abnormal. The Huntington's gene codes for glutamine, so the expansion produces a long polyglutamine which interacts with other cellular proteins, causing toxicity and death. The age of onset and possibly the rate of disease progression are thought to relate to the length of the repeat sequence. In subsequent generations the number of repeats can increase, producing earlier manifestation. This is called anticipation.

In Friedreich's ataxia a GAA repeat has been identified in gene X15 at 9q13–q21.1. In fragile X syndrome CGG repeats on the X chromosome (at Xq27.3) cause inactivation of the gene and also cause the chromosome to break more easily under certain conditions. X-linked spinal and bulbar muscular atrophy (Kennedy's disease) is due to CAG repeats in the SBMA gene at Xq11–12, which codes for the androgen receptor. Spinocerebellar ataxia type I mapps to 6p22–p23 with an expansion of CAG repeats, Dentato–rubro–pallido–luysian atrophy is due to a CAG expansion at 12p12–ter. Marchado–Joseph disease is due to a CAG expansion at 14q24.3–q32.

Myoclonus – brief shock-like muscular jerk
Tremor – rhythmical, repetitive movements
Chorea – sustained writhing movement
Dystonic – sustained abnormal posture
Hemibalismus – violent movements of a limb
Tics – brief twitches, partially under voluntary control

Table 18.3 Involuntary movements

disorders classify all sorts of movements as dystonic, but the most common seen in clinical practice would be either the movements seen with excessive treatment with dopaminergic agents or torticollis (wry neck). Paroxysmal choreoathetosis and dopa responsive dystonia are discussed in Chapter 19.

Idiopathic torsion dystonia

This is the most common idiopathic dystonia and has an incidence of about 250 per million. It can either be generalized or manifest itself as fragments of the full blown syndrome. Such fragments might be torticollis or writers' cramp. It is thought to be transmitted in an autosomal dominant fashion with variable penetrance. Although often a family history is not obtained from the patient, actual examination of relatives may reveal minor movement disorders that have not been brought to attention. The focal fragments can be treated with injections of botulinum toxin. This weakens the muscles injected and is particularly affective in torticollis. Treatment of the generalized disorder is unsatisfactory. Anticholinergics such as benzhexol can be used, but large doses have to be utilized and the side effects may not be tolerated by the patient. Benzodiazepines, tetrabenazine and haloperidol are also used with varying success.

Gilles de la Tourette syndrome

This is an autosomal dominant syndrome with variable penetrance, favouring males. It consists of multiple tics, involuntary vocalizations such as barking or occasionally copralalia and obsessive compulsive behaviour. It has an incidence of 30/100 000 and responds to haloperidol.

Tremor

There is a normal physiological tremor of about 8–12 Hz which can be exaggerated by a number of situations, such as anxiety, drugs or thyrotoxicosis (Table 18.4). Essential tremor (senile tremor) has a frequency of 5–8 Hz and is often associated with a family history. It is

Exaggeration of physiological tremor
Thyrotoxicosis
Alcohol withdrawal
Essential tremor
Drugs (sympathomimetics)
Intention tremor
Cerebellar dysfunction, e.g. MS
Rest tremor
Parkinson's disease
Drug-induced Parkinsonism

Table 18.4 Types of tremor

often suppressed by two units of alcohol for up to an hour. Propanolol can also suppress the tremor with less in the way of deleterious social consequences. Primary orthostatic tremor is discussed in Chapter 19.

Neuroleptic-induced movement disorders

Neuroleptics are powerful drugs and given the incidence of psychiatric illness it is not surprising that the side effects of these drugs are frequently encountered. There are three main neurological complications, drug-induced Parkinsonism, neuroleptic malignant syndrome (NMS) and tarditive dyskinesia (TD). NMS is discussed in chapter 19.

The neuroleptics block dopamine receptors, so on occasion inducing the cardinal features of Parkinson's disease, tremor, bradykinesia and rigidity. The features often only present while the patient is taking neuroleptics and the patient returns to normal on discontinuation of treatment within a few days to weeks. It may be that the neuroleptics have made manifest an underlying Parkinsonian tendency, in which case there may be no return to normality. There is then a therapeutic dilemma as anti-Parkinsonian drugs will tend to worsen the psychiatric state. Sulparide and clozapine are purported to be the least Parkinsonian of the major tranquillizers.

Tarditive dyskinesia is seen in about a fifth of patients on long-term neuroleptic treatment. It consists of lip-smacking and tongue protrusion with rocking of the trunk, and in more florid cases, choreiform movements of the limbs. Tarditive dyskinesia is thought to be a result of super-sensitization of dopamine receptors after years of blockade. It often gets worse on discontinuing the phenothiazines and paradoxically may be suppressed for a while on increasing the dose. In two-thirds of patients the condition remits over the 3 years following drug withdrawal. It is resistant to treatment, but high dose anticholinergics have a limited role.

MCQs for Chapter 18

The MCQs are either true T or false F. The answers are given in Appendix 3. Negatively mark your answers; a point for a correct answer, deduct a point for an incorrect response. If you score 24 or more you pass.

1. **The cardinal features of Parkinson's disease are:**
   A Tremor.
   B Bradykinesia.
   C Dystonias.
   D Rigidity.

2. **Causes of Parkinsonism include:**
   A Atherosclerosis.
   B Iodine poisoning.
   C Encephalitis lethargica.
   D Multisystem atrophy.

3. **Parkinson's disease:**
   A The peak age of onset is 40.
   B There is loss of dopaminergic input into the substantia nigra.
   C Pick bodies are pathognomonic of Parkinson's disease.
   D The incidence of Parkinson's disease is about 5/100 000.

4. **Clinical features of Parkinson's disease:**
   A The posture is often stooped.
   B Clasp–knife spasticity is classical.
   C The tremor is worse on intention.
   D Postural reflexes are often impaired.

5. **Drugs used in the treatment of Parkinson's disease include:**
   A Orphenadrine.
   B Selegeline.
   C Chlorpromazine.
   D Metoclopramide.

6.
   A Autonomic failure is a cardinal feature of multisystem atrophy.

   B Impotence is a late symptom in multisystem atrophy.
   C Horizontal gaze is initially affected in progressive supranuclear palsy.
   D Intellectual impairment occurs as progressive supranuclear palsy progresses.

7. **Movement disorders:**
   A Myoclonus is sustained writhing movements.
   B Hemibalismus is violent movements of a limb.
   C Tics are partly under voluntary control.
   D Tremor is a rhythmical repetitive movement.

8.
   A Idiopathic torsion dystonia is autosomal recessive.
   B Botulinum toxin is good at treating generalized dystonia.
   C Low dose of anticholinergics are effective in dystonia.
   D Torticollis can be part of idiopathic torsion dystonia.

9. **Tremor:**
   A Cerebellar tremor is an exaggeration of physiological tremor.
   B Essential tremor is usually worse at rest.
   C Parkinsonian tremor is worse at rest.
   D Thyrotoxic tremor is an exaggeration of physiological tremor.

10. **Neuroleptic induced movement disorders:**
    A Tarditive dyskinesia initially gets worse after cessation of neuroleptics.
    B Neuroleptics can cause tremor, bradykinesia and rigidity.
    C Clozapine is particularly likely to induce an extrapyramidal syndrome.
    D Lip-smacking is typical of drug-induced parkinsonism.

19. Rare but important neurological disorders

Objectives

This chapter covers a number of disparate topics not dealt with in the other chapters. They are:

- Neurosyphilis
- Benign intercranial hypertension
- Normal pressure hydrocephalus
- Colloid cyst of the third ventricle
- Juvenile myoclonic epilepsy
- Slow meningeal processes
- Treatable movement disorders
- Tetanus
- Motor neurone disease

Most of this book has been concerned with either symptoms, common neurological conditions or conceptual issues. This leaves a series of rare but important conditions that need considering. The reason they are included is that it is important to recognize them as they are either treatable or have major prognostic implications for the patients. Necessarily this chapter is a bit of a *pot-pourri*.

General paralysis of the insane
Dementia
Tabes dorsalis
Spinal cord, particularly posterior column
Meningovascular syphilis
Isolated cerebral blood vessels
Isolated cranial nerves

Table 19.1 Tertiary neurosyphilis

Neurosyphilis

Syphilis is supposed to be making a comeback, particularly in male homosexuals, but the late complications remain very rare. Co-infection with HIV shortens the period from primary infection to tertiary syphilis to a few months. Usually it takes years to decades for the three forms of tertiary neurosyphilis to develop (Table 19.2).

Syphilis had the reputation for being able to manifest itself with any neurological symptom. A few decades ago it would have been impossible to pass through a neurological department without having a WR (serological test for syphilis) performed.

In neurosyphilis, as well as a positive blood FTA and usually a positive blood VDRL in the CSF, there will be an elevated protein, oligoclonal bands, a lymphocytic pleocytosis and often though not invariably, a positive VDRL. Nowadays health economics analysis tends to discourage the random testing though testing is still part of antenatal care. Meningovascular syphilis responds to treatment. GPI and tabes generally do not and there may be an exacerbation of symptoms on treatment (Herxhiemer reaction) which can be limited by concurrent steroid coverage.

Benign intercranial hypertension (BIH)

This is a condition that usually affects obese young females. Other precipitants are given in Table 19.2. BIH consists of raised intracranial pressure with no mass present. Its old name was pseudotumour cerebri. The clinical features are those of headache, nausea and vomiting. Papilloedema is almost always present. Visual obscurations may occur and they are an important warning of incipient blindness which may be permanent. Usually the ventricles are small on CT. The CSF opening pressure is elevated, often spectacularly, but the CSF is otherwise normal. The normal CSF pressure at lumbar puncture is quoted as being less than 25 cm of CSF. Most patients have pressures in the 5–15 range and an opening pressure of 20 or over should not exclude the diagnosis of BIH if all the other features are present. BIH has to be differentiated from cerebral venous sinus thrombosis (see Chapter 15). This can be done by looking at the venous phase of cerebral angiography or doing an MRI to look at the venous sinuses. Emergency treatment and diagnosis are achieved by doing the LP. Treatment with 250 mg acetazolamide two or three times a day is usually sufficient. Sometimes a thiazide is used instead. The underlying cause needs addressing. This

usually consists of gradual but steady weight loss. If medical treatment fails then the choice is between optic nerve fenestration and ventricular or lumbar shunt insertion.

Normal pressure hydrocephalus (NPH)

This presents with the triad of gait apraxia, urinary incontinence and dementia. There is radiological evidence for a communicating hydrocephalus with enlarged ventricles, but the CSF pressure measured at lumbar puncture is normal. As it is a disease of older patients there are major difficulties in differentiating it from the other dementias, particularly as brain atrophy not infrequently results in enlargement of the ventricles. When ventricular enlargement is secondary to loss of brain parenchyma it is called ex-vacuuol. Sulcal and Sylvian fissure widening are radiological clues that the process is ex-vacuuol rather than hydrocephalic, but often it is impossible to tell. Prolonged intracranial pressure monitoring can detect waves of high pressure in NPH. An alternative strategy is to assess the mental state and walking in a quantitative fashion and then to do daily lumbar punctures for 5 days. If there is an improvement then that is reasonable evidence to recommend shunt insertion for treatment of presumed NPH.

Colloid cyst of the third ventricle

This is an extraordinarily rare but treatable cause of headache. If a colloid cyst lies in the third ventricle it may interfere with the drainage of CSF, resulting in an intermittent hydrocephalus. This produces headache and vomiting, which may be intermittent and, on close questioning, positional. It would be all too easy to dismiss such headaches as migraine or tension-type headaches and in the one case I have diagnosed I did. Fortuitously I did a CT scan which demonstrated the lesion and the

Tetracycline
Corticosteroids, either usage or discontinuation
Combined oral contraceptive pill
Vitamin A
Ear infections
Weight gain

Table 19.2 Factors that can precipitate BIH

hydrocephalus. Treatment is surgical with either removal of the cyst or shunting.

Juvenile myoclonic epilepsy

This epileptic syndrome is important because the treatment is effective and specific. Its onset is usually in the 12–18-year age group. Twenty-five per cent of patients will have a family history. Patients have myoclonic jerks first thing in the morning. Often these jerks have been ignored and have to be specifically questioned for. It is the associated generalized seizures that bring the patient to medical attention. These respond very well to sodium valproate, but may worsen with other anti-epileptics. The EEG demonstrates polyspike and spike and wave activity at a higher frequency than 3 Hz.

Slow meningeal processes

One of the reoccurring diagnostic challenges is that of a patient with a progressive neurological disorder attributable to mischief in the subarachnoid space. This can present with pain, multiple cranial nerve palsies or radiculopathies. The spinal fluid is abnormal with a raised protein and lymphocytes with or without a few polymorphs. There is a list of 'funnies' that should be considered under these circumstances (Table 19.3), but the most common 'funny' is lymphoma.

Lymphoma, carcinoma, lysteria, cryptococcus, tuberculosis and Lyme disease have been previously discussed in Chapter 11. Myco-

plasma, while being primarily a lung infection not infrequently has neurological complications. The exact mechanism of their production is not clear but a circulating neurotoxin is a leading contender. As well as multiple radiculopathies and a lymphocytic CSF an encephalopathy can be encountered which can be complicated by seizure activity.

Neurosarcoid can be difficult to diagnose. As well as parenchymal lesions granulomata can form along the leptomeninges, causing multiple cranial neuropathies, the most common being a VIIth palsy. Often there is no spread outside the CNS so the serum angiotensin-converting enzyme level may not be raised. There may be no extracranial deposits at biopsy. Under these circumstances either leptomeningeal biopsy or the Kveim test can be useful. Treatment is with long courses of corticosteroids.

Treatable movement disorders

These movement disorders may be rare, but they are very rewarding to diagnose as they are treatable.

Wilson's disease

Wilson's disease is an autosomal recessive disorder of copper metabolism with a failure to excrete the metal in the bile resulting in toxic accumulations in the liver and brain. It has a reported incidence of 30 per million. Forty per cent of patients present with neurological symptoms such as an akinetic rigidity, dystonia or pseudocerebellar syndrome. Dystonia of the face can eventually lead to an apparently smiling face – risus sardonicus. Psychiatric presentations occur in 20%. The caeruloplasmin is low in the vast majority of cases and Kayser–Fleischer rings can be seen on slit-lamp examination. Urinary copper excretion is elevated, but liver biopsy for liver copper levels is necessary in some cases. All patients who present under 50 years of age with a movement disorder need to have this diagnosis considered as if left untreated it is

Lymphoma
Carcinoma
Lysteria
Mycoplasma
Cryptococcus
Tuberculosis
Lyme disease
Sarcoid

Table 19.3 Slow meningeal processes

fatal. It has been estimated that half of the cases of Wilson's disease in the UK are failing to be diagnosed. Therapy is d-penicillamine which increases the urinary excretion of copper.

Dopa-responsive dystonia

Most forms of generalized dystonia are poorly responsive to treatment; however, there is a subset that respond well to L-dopa. Onset is within the first two decades of life. Patients present as a dystonia with or without Parkinsonian features. There tends to be diurnal variation initially, often with a spastic diplegia with brisk reflexes and extensor plantar responses. Dopa-responsive dystonia is inherited in a dominant fashion with incomplete penetrance. All patients with onset of generalized dystonia in the first half of life should be tried on L-dopa, initially at low doses but building up to 250 mg three times a day for 3 months prior to deciding if there is no response.

Paroxysmal kinesogenic choreoathetosis

This condition is autosomally inherited in two-thirds of cases with onset in childhood or adolescence. On moving, such as standing up, episodes of choreoathetosis are induced. These attacks last less than 5 minutes, but may occur many times a day. They respond very well to either carbamazepine or phenytoin.

Primary orthostatic tremor

This tremor develops on standing. It can be due to cerebellar disease, action myoclonus or essential tremor. After a few seconds of standing the patient develops a 16 Hz tremor in the legs. This is often interpreted by the patient as unsteadiness on standing. Clonazepam can often be helpful.

Restless legs syndrome

Restless legs syndrome is a common disorder occurring in about 0.5% of the population. It is present during the day, but at night can severely disrupt sleep. It is characterized by an annoying aching, crawling sensation predominantly affecting the legs. It can be associated with uraemia, iron deficiency or chronic ethanol use. It is often familial and it responds to clonazepam or fluoxetine.

Oculogyric crisis

This is usually a complication of dopamine-blocking drugs such as phenothiazines or other major tranquillizers, but many antinausea medications, such as metoclopramide, can precipitate attacks. The patient develops an acute dystonia which is often heralded by forced up gaze of the eyes and then goes on to involve the jaw and limbs with arching of the back. When this condition develops unexpectedly it sends the patient and their attendant medical staff into a state of total panic. The offending medication should be stopped, but for acute therapy a very gratifying response to 5 mg procyclidine or diazepam intravenously can be obtained.

Neuroleptic malignant syndrome (NMS) and malignant hyperpyrexia (MH)

These two separate conditions share some features in common. Neuroleptic malignant syndrome is precipitated by neuroleptics or rarely antidepressants. Malignant hyperpyrexia is precipitated by anaesthetic agents such as suxamethonium or halothane. It is often autosomally dominantly inherited. Both conditions are characterized by stiffness in the muscles and fever. MH has a hyperacute course and treatment is with dantroline sodium given intravenously. NMS develops over several days and is treated with bromocriptine or dantroline. Both are associated with high creatine kinase levels in the blood. In the past both were associated with a high mortality.

Tetanus

Tetanus is rare in countries with a developed immunization programme and as such most clinicians have no experience of it. It is due to infection of a wound with *Clostridium tetani* which is a ubiquitous organism found in soil and faeces, particularly of the horse. Patients who sustain a wound likely to be infected with *Cl. tetani* should receive penicillin and in high risk cases (unimmunized) receive antitetanus immunoglobulin. Often there is co-infection of the wound with other organisms, or a foreign body present. After an incubation period of a week neurotoxin initially causes local muscular spasms, followed by widespread pain and muscular spasm. The neurotoxin blocks inhibition of α-motor neurones. In the head it causes trismus and risus sardonicus. The neck is extended and opisthotonic spasms of the spine occur. Death is from asphyxia or cardiac arrest. The mortality used to be over 80%, but with modern intensive care facilities it is about 30%.

Motor neurone disease (MND)/ amyotrophic lateral sclerosis (ALS)

MND is a grim disease with an incidence of 0.4 to 1.8 per 100 000. The Americans call it ALS or more picturesquely Lou Garric's disease. Lou Garric was one of the all time great baseball players who was struck down with ALS. One of the most moving clips of film I have ever seen is his final address to his fans where he says what a wonderful life he has had. MND was described by Charcot between 1865 and 1874. In its classical form it consists of a combination of upper and lower motor neurone signs and symptoms. The aetiology is unknown, but 5–10% of cases are familial in an autosomal dominant fashion. There is no clinical sensory involvement. It is usually relentlessly progressive with 50% dead within 3 years from onset. The earlier the age of onset, the longer the survival. Cases of survival of up to 20 years have been reported, but one wonders if that is the same disease and certainly diagnostic confusion can arise with the spinal muscular atrophies and multifocal motor neuropathy with conduction block (see

Chapter 13). The diagnosis is primarily clinical, but there are some pitfalls to be aware of (Table 19.4) As the diagnosis is a death sentence more than usual care must be taken in making it. The usual presentation is of progressive painless weakness in a limb or progressive bulbar problems in a middle-aged person. On examination the weakness is usually more widespread than the patient appreciated, diffuse fasciculations and wasting can be seen. Hyper-reflexia and extensor plantar responses may be present. If the tongue is affected there may be observable atrophy and fasciculations. While a very useful clinical sign, as it demonstrates pathology above the foramen magnum, it is difficult to observe. The tongue has to lie in the floor of the mouth in a relaxed state. Most patients find this difficult to do. In the presence of the classical findings a routine biochemical screen including glucose and creatine kinase, thyroid function tests and electrophysiological examination are often sufficient. Many neurologists would include acetylcholine receptor antibody titres and cervical cord imaging. The usefulness of the electrophysiological examination is dependent on the skill of the electrophysiologist. Motor conduction block should be specifically sought as its presence would change the diagnosis.

Motor neurone disease-like syndromes
Dysproteinaemia
Thyroid dysfunction
Vitamin B_{12} deficiency
Vasculitis
Lead toxicity
Hexosaminidase A deficiency
Prior poliomyelitis
Other diagnostic traps
Lesions at the foramen magnum
Cervical spondylotic myeloradiculopathy
Cervical and high thoracic cord tumours
Diabetic amyotrophy
Chronic inflammatory demyelinating polyneuropathy
Multifocal conduction block
Myasthenia gravis
Lambert–Eaton myasthenic syndrome

Table 19.4 The differential diagnosis of motor neurone disease

Case history

Freda Talke was a 65-year-old retired district nurse who tripped while shopping and subsequently noticed her right foot was not working properly. Her daughter, who was a physiotherapist, brought her to see me. On examination there was a right foot drop. The reflexes were a bit brisk, but nothing else was abnormal. A presumptive diagnosis of a lacunar infarct was made and she underwent the usual investigations including a CT scan of the head, all of which were normal. Her daughter brought her back to see me 3 months later. Far from the leg getting better Mrs Talke thought it had actually deteriorated. On examination most of the muscles in the right leg were a bit weak, the plantar response was extensor and there was mild weakness of dorsiflexion in the left foot. A creatine kinase was normal as was a cervical MRI. An electrophysiological examination was not diagnostic. On review a further 3 months later she had a slight but definite slurring of the speech and there was some weakness of right shoulder abduction. A presumptive diagnosis of motor neurone disease was made. A further electrophysiological examination was performed which showed evidence of denervation in all four limbs and at review 3 months later sparse fasciculations could be seen in all four limbs. Within a further 6 months she was having difficulty making herself understood and had difficulty swallowing. She could just walk with two sticks. She had tremendous support from her family and required a gastrostomy tube to be inserted 2 months later. At that time she could not swallow her own saliva, she was wheelchair bound and was losing the use of her arms. Mercifully she died within a couple of weeks from respiratory failure secondary to a chest infection.

Care of the motor neurone disease patient should be multidisciplinary. Initial denial or depression is not unusual and may necessitate counselling. The MND society have useful literature and can often provide support. The team should include physiotherapists, speech therapists, occupational therapists, social workers, neurologists and general practitioners.

Percutaneous endoscopic gastrostomy is useful for nutritional support. Decisions about the appropriateness of ventilatory support need to be taken before a crisis occurs. Opiates are very useful for respiratory distress.

Riluzol at a dose of 50 mg b.d. has been demonstrated to prologue the course of the disease. While inappropriate for patients in the later stages of the illness it should be offered to patients with early disease in the hope of prolonging useful life.

MCQs for Chapter 19

The MCQs are either true T or false F. The answers are given in Appendix 3. Negatively mark your answers; a point for a correct answer, deduct a point for an incorrect response. If you score 24 or more you pass.

1. **Neurosyphilis:**
   A Oligoclonal bands are present in neurosyphilis.
   B Treatment of general paralysis of the insane may exacerbate symptoms.
   C Tabes dorsalis causes an irreversible dementia.
   D Co-infection with HIV delays the development of tertiary syphilis.

2. **Precipitants of benign intracranial pressure include:**
   A Obesity.
   B Acetazolamide.
   C Tetracyclines.
   D Climbing at altitude.

3. **The cardinal features of normal pressure hydrocephalus are:**
   A A non-communicating hydrocephalus.
   B Urinary incontinence.
   C Gait apraxia.
   D Dementia.

4.
   A Juvenile myoclonic epilepsy responds well to carbamazepine.
   B Myoclonic jerks typically occur at night in juvenile myoclonic epilepsy.
   C Restless legs syndrome can be associated with uraemia.
   D Restless legs syndrome occurs in about 1/100 000 of the population.

5. **The following produce a slow meningeal process:**
   A Lymphoma.
   B Pneumococcus.
   C Cryptococcus.
   D Amyloid.

6.
   A Caeruloplasmin levels are high in Wilson's disease.
   B Dopa-responsive dystonia usually presents in the fifth decade.
   C Paroxysmal kinesogenic choreoathetosis responds to carbamazepine.
   D Oculogyric crisis responds to procyclidine.

7.
   A Malignant hyperpyrexia can be precipitated by halothane.
   B Malignant hyperpyrexia is inherited in an autosomal dominant fashion.
   C Neuroleptic malignant syndrome responds to haloperidol.
   D Neuroleptic malignant syndrome and malignant hyperpyrexia cause hypotonia.

8. **Tetanus:**
   A The causative organism is rare in temperate countries.
   B The incubation period can be up to 6 months.
   C The neurotoxin blocks inhibition of the α-motor neurone.
   D Death is from asphyxia or cardiac arrest.

9. **Motor neurone disease:**
   A Has an incidence of approximately 1/100 000.
   B 50% of patients with motor neurone disease are dead within 3 years.
   C Sensory symptoms are occasionally prominent.
   D Extensor plantar responses are rare.

10. **Conditions that can mimic motor neurone disease include:**
    A Lesions at the foramen magnum.
    B Diabetic amyotrophy.
    C Thyrotoxicosis.
    D Multifocal conduction block.

20. Neurological emergencies

Objectives

The following neurological emergencies will be discussed:

- Status epilepticus
- Coma
- Acute cord compression
- Subarachnoid haemorrhage
- Stroke in evolution
- Neuromuscular respiratory failure
- Herniation
- Bacterial meningitis

The neurological emergencies are those neurological conditions that can evolve rapidly and where intervention can reduce mortality and morbidity. For some reason they often occur late on Friday afternoon or at 2 o'clock in the morning. It is useful for every clinician to understand these disorders and their initial management as neurological expertise may not be immediately available, though it should never be more than a telephone call away. The neurological emergencies are also great fun to manage as in fact if one follows a few simple rules there is a logical course of action in each case. It is likely that other medical staff, nursing staff, the relatives and the patient themselves will be in a state of high anxiety. Someone who knows what they are doing relieves everyone else's stress and can rapidly restore effectiveness to the team, as well as potentially saving lives and avoiding long-term disability, to bastardize Kipling, 'if you can keep your head while all around are losing theirs, you'll be a neurologist friend'.

Status epilepticus (convulsive)

Status epilepticus is defined as constant tonic-clonic seizures for 30 minutes or seizures so frequent that normal consciousness is not retained between fits. While initially the blood pressure is elevated, after about half an hour it starts to fall. In addition, respiration is often embarrassed. Hyperpyrexia, hypoglycaemia and reflex pulmonary oedema can develop. Because of the seizure activity the metabolic rate of the brain is high, but the means to support that high metabolic rate are compromised, so eventually permanent brain damage will result. If the status is allowed to continue for more than an hour the likelihood of permanent damage rises. Therefore the aim of treatment should be to have status broken within an hour. The mortality is between 5 and 25%.

It is not a diagnosis. A cause should be sought and treated appropriately. While the most common cause of status is a known epileptic having forgotten to take their medication, optimal management of the status will be to no avail if an underlying bacterial meningitis is not appreciated.

The two major errors frequently seen in the management of status are incorrect diagnosis and the use of homeopathic doses of anti-epileptic drugs (AEDs). Non-epileptic seizure disorder (pseudo-status) should be briefly considered before embarking on aggressive and potentially harmful regimens of AEDs. NESD is discussed in Chapter 16. It can present as status, which is resistant to AEDs. Clues to a diagnosis of non-epileptic status are directed violence, forced eye closure and shaking of the head from side to side, but EEG may be required to be certain. If the diagnosis is not appreciated more and more AEDs are given until the patient becomes respiratorally embarrassed and ends up on an intensive care unit sedated and ventilated. While this does stop NESD status, it is neither a cost-effective or a particularly safe management plan.

On finding a patient in status the first thing to do is the standard resuscitation checklist of airway, breathing and output. Plastic airways can be used, but other objects such as fingers or spoons should not be put between the teeth. The former may get bitten off while the latter may break teeth. Intravenous access should be obtained and blood drawn for the investigations in Table 20.1. Not all of these will always be appropriate, but they all should be considered. A blood glucose estimation on a BM

stick should be performed at the same time. Thiamine and glucose should be given to patients arriving off the street. The second most common precipitant of status is alcohol and if the patient is thiamine deficient a glucose load could precipitate Wernicke's encephalopathy. A bolus of 5–20 mg of intravenous diazepam will often terminate status. Care has to be given to its respiratory depressant effect. As an intravenous bolus it is very effective, but within a minute or two the diazepam will have been redistributed and no longer be an effective anticonvulsant. If the patient has a tendency to go back into status then another AED will be required. Although no longer a first line, oral AED phenytoin is potent and, used appropriately, an effective AED in status. The loading dose is large and often physicians are too timid and give too little. With a loading dose of 20 mg/kg an average male of 70 kg will require 1.4 g! If the patient is not already on phenytoin I start with 1 g, knowing I can safely give a further 500 mg if status continues. If the patient is already on phenytoin I give 500 mg. The phenytoin should be given intravenously over half to three-quarters of an hour with cardiac monitoring. Phenytoin is arrhythmogenic and a negative inotrope if given as a bolus. The patient will then need an additional 300 mg a day maintenance dose. In the vast majority of patients with status this is all that will be needed. If this fails then it is worth reconsidering the diagnosis or the underlying brain pathology. The next drug depends on local familiarity. Many people use chlomethiazole, but it has dangerous kinetics on continued administration resulting in prolonged sedation or coma. It comes in a 0.8% solution. An initial 50 ml is given over 10 minutes and then a continuous infusion of about 0.5 ml an hour is given which is titrated against the patient's level of arousal and seizures. An alternative is to use intravenous valproate with a loading dose of 400–800 mg over 5 minutes. This seems remarkably free of side effects and as we get more experience it may take the place of phenytoin. If the patient continues in status despite the above medications then there is a problem. The patient

---

1. **A**irway **B**reathing **C**irculation
2. IV access – bloods for:
   FBC
   U&E
   Glucose
   Calcium and magnesium
   Toxicology/drug levels
   BM stick
3. i.v. 50 ml of 50% dextrose and 100 mg thiamine
4. Diazepam 5–20 mg i.v.
5. Phenytoin 20 mg/kg over $\frac{1}{2}$ hr with cardiac monitoring or valproate 400–800 mg i.v. over 5 min
6. Phenobarbital 10 mg/kg twice with respiratory support
7. Ventilate, paralyse and add more barbiturates

Table 20.1 Management of status epilepticus

should be moved to an intensive care setting with respiratory support available and phenobarbitone should be given. Again the loading dose is large. If this fails the patient should be ventilated and sufficient barbiturates given to suppress seizure activity. EEG monitoring will be required to determine the electrical state of the brain as the physical manifestations of the seizures will be absent if paralysing drugs have been used. Often a burst suppression pattern is seen under these circumstances with bursts of seizure activity interspersed with flat line EEG. This has a poor prognosis. I have seen it in anoxic encephalopathy and carcinomatous meningitis.

Status epilepticus partialis continua

If there is a focal cause for the epilepsy then a focal status epilepticus can develop. This can be simple with no clouding of consciousness or there may be some interference with normal thinking. It is less life-threatening than generalized status, but can itself generalize. At times it can be quite resistant to treatment. The same drugs as in generalized status can be used as well as oral medications. The underlying cause will need to be determined and treated if appropriate (e.g. cerebral abscess).

Non-convulsive status

In non-convulsive status there is generalized abnormal electrical activity, but no tonic-clonic limb movements. This can present as a confusional state or apparently psychiatric state. The difficulty is considering the diagnosis as the vast majority of confusional states are not due to non-convulsive status. Usually there is a past history of epilepsy, or a few tonic-clonic seizures in association. A pseudo-non-convulsive status not infrequently occurs in intensive care where neuromuscular blocking agents may mask the tonic-clonic manifestations of epilepsy. An EEG can be invaluable in an ITU patient who is not recovering neurologically as if status is demonstrated then therapy can improve the outcome.

Coma

'death like sleep might steal on me' (Percy Bysshe Shelly 1792–1822)

Consciousness is the most important aspect of existence. Loss of consciousness implies a catastrophic failure of homeostasis and is often a harbinger of death. The level of consciousness will correlate with the severity of the situation. The timely assessment and management of the comatose patient is a critical clinical skill.

The most common cause of coma of unknown aetiology is drug poisoning (30%). This is included in the 65% with diffuse or metabolic causes of their coma, where a CT scan of the head will be non-diagnostic. So it is illogical to rush to CT scanning as an initial investigation. As with all critical patients the ABC of resuscitation has to be the first step. The intravenous access has to be obtained and blood drawn for the investigations listed in Table 20.2. Not all those investigations will be required on all patients. The blood gases

DON'T PANIC
1. Assess respiratory and cardiovascular status (**ABC**)
2. Intravenous access
3. Bloods:　　　　Glucose
　　　　　　　　Electrolytes
　　　　　　　　Urea creatinine
　　　　　　　　LFT
　　　　　　　　Full blood count
　　　　　　　　Clotting studies
　　　　　　　　Tox screen and drug levels
　　　　　　　　B.M. stick
　　　　　　　　Gases
4. Thiamine 100 mg i.v., dextrose 50 ml 50% i.v. and naloxone 0.8 mg i.v.
5. History; ambulance personnel, work mates, family
6. Examination:　Level of consciousness (GCS)
　　　　　　　　Brain-stem reflexes
　　　　　　　　Signs of trauma (Battle's sign, Raccoon sign)
　　　　　　　　Skin (rashes, jaundice, track marks)
　　　　　　　　Infection (fever, neck stiffness)
　　　　　　　　Localizing neurological signs
7. Non-contrast CT scan if stable
8. Spinal tap if indicated

Table 20.2 The emergency room assessment of coma

Metabolic
  Glucose
  Hypoxic/hypoperfusion
  Hepatic failure
  Renal failure
Toxic
  Iatrogenic (benzodiazepines, opiates)
  OD (tricyclics, opiates, barbiturates)
Bicerebral (or one hemisphere with mass effect)
Brain stem – reticular activating system
Psychogenic

Table 20.3 Differential diagnosis of coma

Descriptions of the level of consciousness
Awake and alert – attends to environment spontaneously
Drowsy – tendency not to attend to environment
Stuporous – needs constant stimulation in order to attend
Comatose – cannot attend to environment

Glasgow Coma Scale

Best eye opening response:	
spontaneous	4
to speech	3
to pain	2
none	1
Best verbal response:	
oriented	5
confused conversation	4
short inappropriate exclamations	3
incomprehensible moans/groans	2
none	1
Best motor response:	
obeys verbal commands	6
localizes painful stimulus	5
limb flexion in response to pain	4
flexion abnormality (decorticate)	3
limb extension in response to pain (decerebrate)	2
none	1
	[ ]

The GCS is generous; you score 3 if you are dead.

Table 20.4 Assessment of level of consciousness

will require a separate arterial stick, and are extremely useful in that they give information not only on oxygenation, but also CO_2 retention and acid-base status. The cocktail of thiamine, dextrose and naloxone should be given to anyone brought in from the street. The thiamine is to stop the development of Wernicke's encephalopathy in alcoholics, the glucose is to reverse hypoglycaemic coma and the naloxone reverses opiates. The usual source of a history is unavailable, but that makes any source of information all the more valuable. The differential diagnosis of coma is wide (Table 20.3) and any clue is a great help. The examination should document the level of coma. This can either be done in English or for the linguistically challenged with the Glasgow Coma Scale (Table 20.4). It does not matter as long as the next person reading the notes has an accurate picture of the patient's condition at that time. The brain-stem reflexes (Chapter 11) are important to record as their loss has poor prognostic implications. Evidence for trauma has to be sought. Running gloved hands through the hair will often reveal lacerations to the scalp. Battle's sign is subcutaneous haemorrhage behind the ear, Raccoon's sign is a black eye without direct eye trauma. They are both signs of skull fracture and can take a few days to develop. Blood in the external auditory meatus (ear) can also indicate a base of skull fracture. If there is a possibility of head trauma care must be taken in manipulating the neck as a concomitant neck injury has to be presumed.

After initial resuscitation, and while the laboratory is analysing the blood tests, it may be appropriate to obtain a non-contrast CT of the head. The patient has to be stable as they will not be monitored as closely in the CT scanner as in the resuscitation area. If the CT scan does not demonstrate the potential for herniation then occasionally a lumbar puncture will be required. This is primarily to look for meningitis, as a subarachnoid haemorrhage large enough to render someone unconscious for any period of time would be demonstrable on CT.

There are situations which may be mistaken for coma. This is why it is a good policy never to discuss patients in their presence as if they are not there and to explain who you are and what you are doing. The four situations are locked in syndrome, top of the basilar syndrome, motor nerve or neuromusclar junction failure, and psychiatric unresponsiveness.

Locked in syndrome

Ventral lesions of the pons (haemorrhage, pontine myelinolysis, infarcts) result in de-efferentation of the patient. The patient is unresponsive, but awake and receiving sensory input. The only voluntary movement may be vertical eye movements.

Top of the basilar syndrome

Emboli lodging at the bifurcation of the basilar can cause an infarction in the upper brain stem and possibly occipital lobes. The patient may have bilateral ptosis and be drowsy, but is in fact rousable.

Disorders of the neuromuscular junction or motor nerves

As the only way we communicate with the external world is via muscular action any disease which sufficiently impairs muscular function can make a patient unresponsive. On occasion myasthenia, Guillain–Barré and botulism can give this appearance.

Psychiatric coma

One could argue as to whether psychiatric disorders truly lead to coma. They account for 1.5% of cases of coma of unknown aetiology and are due to conversion reactions, depression and catatonic stupor.

Acute cord compression

Cord disease is discussed in Chapter 12. Here we will concentrate on acute, non-traumatic cord compression. It is a neurological emergency because the final events often become ischaemic so quickly and irreversible and the patient is left in a wheelchair, incontinent of urine and faeces. The most common cause of acute cord compression is metastatic disease. The difficulty is considering the diagnosis. Once the possibility has been recognized investigation of the patient is mandatory. The most

Case history

John Bradley was admitted as an emergency having been found collapsed at home. He was a 35-year-old ex-alcoholic who smoked 30 cigarettes a day. His family had become concerned when he had not come down to breakfast on the Sunday morning. On examination he was unrousable, had a tachycardia of 130 and had fixed dilated pupils. The medical team made a diagnosis of a brain-stem stroke and admitted him to the ward. The family were told that the prognosis was grave. Next morning he was sitting up in bed having his breakfast when the post take ward round arrived. It transpired that he had taken an overdose of amitriptyline which had produced the coma, dilated pupils and tachycardia.

important features of cord compression are given in Table 20.5.

The time between presentation and initiation of therapy should be less than 24 hours. The protocol for managing patients with suspected acute cord compression is presented in Table 20.6.

The key factor in this process is the timely imaging of the spinal cord. This used to be done by myelography followed by CT scanning of the area of the block, but nowadays MRI has all but taken over. The disadvantages of myelography are that it is invasive, may worsen the patient's condition, is uncomfortable and labour intensive. The major pitfall with both techniques is failing to image the complete cord. While a sensory level may indicate a level below which the lesion cannot be, the compression is often higher than suggested by

Back pain
Bilateral motor weakness
Sensory level
Hyper-reflexia and Babinski's (beware spinal shock)
Bowel/bladder/sexual dysfunction
Brown–Séquard syndrome

Table 20.5 Most important features of cord compression

History
Examination
If reasonable suspicion of acute cord compression:
1. Dexamethasone 10–50 mg i.v.
2. Bloods: FBC, U&E, LFT, PT
3. Imaging CXR
    Plain spine films (usually a waste of time)
    MRI or myelography
4. Histological confirmation
    CT-guided biopsy
    Open biopsy
5. Therapy
    Dexamethasone and radiotherapy
    Surgical decompression

Table 20.6 Protocol for the management of acute cord compression

Sudden onset severe headache
Nausea and vomiting
Angor animi
Photophobia
Neck stiffness
Decreased level of consciousness

Table 20.7 Cardinal features of SAH

the level. Once the lesion has been identified, if there is a known primary, radiotherapy can be initiated. If there is no known primary then a CT-guided percutaneous biopsy can be undertaken. Once histology is obtained then radiotherapy can be initiated. Occasionally a decompressing surgical intervention is appropriate, either because the lesion is non-neoplastic, benign or non-responsive to radiotherapy. But as most metastatic disease is anterior to the cord and the commonest surgical approach is posterior there is a danger of destabilizing the spinal column. The anterior surgical approach may be appropriate, but in the thoracic cord this will entail a thoracotomy which may be more than many patients can stand.

Subarachnoid haemorrhage (SAH)

This condition is discussed in Chapter 15. Any patient who presents with sudden onset severe headache has had a subarachnoid haemorrhage until proven otherwise.

Most neurological units see a couple of patients a year who have been discharged from a casualty department with an SAH undiagnosed. Apart from wounding professional pride this risks the patient's life. A small SAH is often the harbinger of a big

one. Thirty per cent of patients with an SAH from an aneurysm rebleed within a few weeks. Half of the patients who have an SAH will die in the first month and half the survivors will be left disabled. Apart from sudden onset of severe headache about half the patients lose consciousness, often transiently, and many are nauseated or vomit. Angor animi, the fear of imminent doom, is also often present. Meningeal symptoms, photophobia and neck stiffness, develop due to the irritant effect of blood on the meninges (Table 20.7).

The initial investigation of choice is a CT scan of the head which will be abnormal in 90% of patients with an SAH on the first day, but if performed later has a falling sensitivity. If the CT is negative then an LP has to be performed. This should be delayed until 12 hours after the ictus to allow xanthochromia to develop in order to differentiate SAH blood from a bloody tap.

Patients with proven or suspected SAH should be nursed in a quiet environment. The calcium channel blocker nimodepine reduces mortality and morbidity; the exact mechanism of its action remains unknown. As long as the patient is neurologically intact the blood pressure should be lowered and the pressor response reduced; β-blockade with atenolol is useful to achieve this. If the patient is comatose with raised intracranial pressure then lowering the blood pressure will reduce cerebral perfusion. A dose of 2 mg of diazepam three times a day will take the edge off patients' anxiety (Table 20.8).

Once the diagnosis of SAH is made the cerebral vasculature will need to be imaged. Currently this is performed with conventional angiography, but MR angiography will take over once the resolution is similar to that of

1. Make a diagnosis
   History and examination
   CT
   LP
     Opening pressure
     Cell count
     Xanthochromia
2. Medical management
   Nurse in quiet calm atmosphere
   Nimodepine
   β-blockade
   Benzodiazepines
3. Further investigations
   Conventional angiography
   MRI/MR angiography
4. Treatment
   Surgical intervention
   Embolization
   Radiosurgery (for AVMs)

Table 20.8 Management of SAH

Maintain BP, unless >230/130
Adequately hydrate
Control hyperglycaemia
Control pyrexia
If evolving and no blood on CT
Rx 5000 units heparin then 700–1000/h, maintaining APTT at 2× control
If carotid territory urgent carotid Doppler studies

Table 20.9 Principles of managing a patient with ischaemic stroke in evolution

the conventional method. The timing of surgical intervention is controversial, but my inclination is to it being as early as possible. Between 3 days and 2 weeks spasm can develop in the cerebral vasculature. This has been less of a problem since the advent of nimodepine, but if there is an unclipped aneurysm then it is dangerous to increase the blood pressure to increase cerebral perfusion.

Stroke in evolution

This field is rapidly developing. Neuroprotective agents are in phase III trials at the time of writing and thrombolytic agents have been used in ischaemic stroke with varying results. Even without further development of the field the patient with a developing stroke represents an opportunity for brain-saving intervention. If a patient has an evolving ischaemic stroke, particularly if the vertebrobasilar system is implicated, then it is reasonable to heparinize the patient. Heparinization should also be used in crescendo TIA once aspirin has failed. The principles of managing a patient with stroke in evolution or crescendo TIA are given in Table 20.9. The principles and further management have been discussed in Chapter 15.

Neuromuscular respiratory failure

A number of neurological conditions such as myasthenia gravis, Guillain–Barré syndrome, multiple sclerosis, muscle disease (acid maltase deficiency), poliomyelitis and motor neurone disease can result in respiratory embarrassment. If the patient has a progressive and irreversible disorder, such as motor neurone disease, a decision about the appropriateness of respiratory support should be made prior to a crisis. Unlike respiratory failure due to lung problems the patient has not got the option of driving the bellows harder. Patients with respiratory failure due to neuromuscular disease look remarkably well until just before they have a respiratory arrest. The terminal problem is often a failure to clear the airway which requires the ability to generate a cough. Parameters used to assess patients are given in Table 20.10.

Diaphragmatic weakness can be assessed by measuring the vital capacity with the patient lying and sitting and watching for the abdomen moving out in inspiration. The automatic response of paramedical staff to lie patients down and place an oxygen mask over the face

Blood gases (good till too late)
Counting numbers in one breath
Vital capacity (panic <1 l)
Negative inspiratory force (panic <25 cm of H_2O)

Table 20.10 Parameters used in the assessment of neurological respiratory failure

ICU for observation
Frequent vital capacity assessment
Nothing by mouth if in danger of aspiration
Intubate and ventilate before arrest

Table 20.11 Principles of managing neuromuscular respiratory failure

can convert a struggling patient into a dead one through the two mechanisms of diaphragmatic weakness and CO_2 retention. While it is important to treat the underlying condition where possible and treat chest infections aggressively, if the patient is teetering on the edge there is no point in wasting time, for example titrating doses of pyridostigmine in the case of myasthenia. It is much better to take control of the respiratory problem with intubation and ventilation than have a patient struggling with near asphyxiation. The principles of managing neuromuscular respiratory failure are given in Table 20.11.

Herniation

This topic is covered in detail in Chapter 11. It is sufficient here to reiterate that herniation requires a pressure gradient rather than raised pressure *per se*. Pressure gradients are caused by brain swelling, space-occupying lesions and non-communicating hydrocephalus. Papilloedema is a late and unreliable sign of raised intracranial pressure. The most important features of herniation are deterioration of level of consciousness, dilatation of the pupils and progressive loss of brain-stem reflexes. This is an emergency and the timely use of the treatments outlined in Table 20.12 can be critical.

500 ml of 20% mannitol i.v.
10 mg dexamethasone i.v.
Urinary catheter
Intubate and hyperventilate
CT for neurosurgically remediable lesion

Table 20.12 Management of herniation

Bacterial meningitis

Bacterial meningitis is a cause of potentially avoidable mortality and morbidity. The matter is discussed in Chapter 11. *The prompt administration of appropriate antibiotics can be life-saving* and herein lies a dilemma. Should patients be treated in the community prior to transfer to hospital or await all the appropriate investigations? I think the guiding principle should be, better a live patient than a neat diagnosis confirmed at autopsy. The signs and symptoms of bacterial meningitis are given in Table 20.13, and the full gamut of investigations are given in Table 20.14.

In adults penicillin G $3–4 \times 10^6$ units i.v. 4-hourly is a good guess for initial therapy in the community. In hospital a cephalosporin is more likely to be used. In children, wider spectrum antibiotics are needed. In addition, volume replacement and pressors may be needed. Adrenocorticosteroids should be used if the patient is shocked. In children it has been demonstrated that steroids reduce the incidence of deafness in survivors.

Fever
Headache
Photophobia
Neck stiffness
Characteristic rash (petechial or purpuric)
Impairment of consciousness
Convulsions
Kernig's sign

Table 20.13 Signs and symptoms of bacterial meningitis

FBC
U&E glucose
Blood cultures at least three
CT (if available)
LP
    Opening pressure
    Cell count
    Protein and glucose
    Gram stain
    Culture
    In selected cases
    Countercurrent electrophoresis
    PCR

Table 20.14 Investigations in bacterial meningitis

MCQs for Chapter 20

The MCQs are either true T or false F. The answers are given in Appendix 3. Negatively mark your answers; a point for a correct answer, deduct a point for an incorrect response. If you score 24 or more you pass.

1. **Status epilepticus:**
   A The most common cause is an epileptic having failed to take their medication.
   B Blood pressure is initially low, but rises in status.
   C The brain's metabolic rate is below normal in status.
   D Pulmonary oedema is a complication.

2. **Drugs used in status epilepticus:**
   A Phenytoin's loading dose is 20 mg/kg.
   B Carbamazepine is a first line alternative.
   C Chlormethiazole is given as a continuous infusion.
   D Cardiac monitoring is required when giving valproate.

3. **Coma:**
   A The most common cause of coma of unknown aetiology is drug poisoning.
   B Naloxone helps prevent Wernicke's encephalopathy.
   C A CT scan of the head will usually identify the cause of coma.
   D In locked in syndrome the patient is unresponsive but awake.

4. **The cardinal features of cord compression include:**
   A Back pain.
   B Fasciculations.
   C Sensory level.
   D Confusion.

5. **The management of cord compression:**
   A Plain spine films usually give a definitive answer.
   B Dexamethasone in high dosage is used.
   C Histology can be obtained by CT-guided biopsy.
   D Most metastatic disease lies posterior to the cord.

6. **Cardinal features of subarachnoid haemorrhage include:**
   A Angor animi.
   B Nausea and vomiting.
   C Unilateral headache.
   D Fortification spectra.

7. **The management of subarachnoid haemorrhage includes:**
   A β-blockade.
   B Subcutaneous heparin.
   C Nimodipine.
   D Broad spectrum antibiotics.

8. **In stroke in evolution:**
   A The blood pressure should rapidly be reduced to 120/70.
   B Patients should be adequately hydrated.
   C Haemorrhage can be confidently excluded on clinical grounds.
   D Hyperglycaemia should be controlled.

9. **Sensitive indicators of incipient neuromuscular respiratory failure are:**
   A Blood gases.
   B Respiratory rate.
   C Vital capacity.
   D Negative inspiratory force.

10. **Signs of bacterial meningitis include:**
    A Convulsions.
    B Kernig's sign.
    C Aching in the limbs.
    D A vesicular rash.

Appendix 1 – The neurological examination

The neurological examination is like sex; it is a practical skill. While reading about it may provide some ideas and be amusing in itself nothing beats actually doing it and to get proficient, doing it repeatedly.

Taking a good history is the most important aspect of making a diagnosis; however, the neurological examination can be contributory and it takes a disproportionate role in clinical examinations. During the process of taking a history various hypotheses have been set up. One of the most important aspects of the examination is to test these hypotheses, both to gather evidence in support or to look for conflicting signs. Because of this aspect of the examination a different examination will be done on nearly every patient. For example, if a hemispheric lesion is suspected the sensory examination of the hands will tend to compare the two hands, while if carpal tunnel syndrome is the presumptive diagnosis the medial and lateral fingers will be compared. This is called a focused examination. At times only a focused examination will be performed; however, when learning clinical skills and when initially meeting a patient there are many advantages in doing a full examination. This involves an element of screening. The reason for doing the screening part of the examination is partly tradition and partly to have a baseline to compare with later; rarely it will find an unexpected abnormality and importantly it conveys to the patient that they are being taken seriously.

The examination consists of a general examination and an assessment of higher mental functions, cranial nerves, limbs, reflexes and gait. A summary of the examination is given in Table A1.1. There is probably little value in reading this appendix as it is. It would be much more useful to go through the examination on a colleague, using this appendix as a guide.

General physical examination

A general examination will frequently give clues as to the diagnosis. How complete it needs to be depends on the circumstances and the presumptive diagnosis. However, the basics of temperature, blood pressure, heart sounds and carotid bruits should be recorded in the vast majority of patients. The heart is important as its malfunction can impact on the brain. In particular, murmurs might indicate a source of emboli as might atrial fibrillation. Hypertension is one of the most important risk factors for stroke. I find it amazing how many patients are assessed for syncope without lying and standing blood pressures being recorded. These simple, inexpensive things will change the whole way a patient will be investigated.

Higher mental functions

It is important to have some assessment of higher cognitive functions for three reasons. First, their dysfunction will have to be incorporated in any pathophysiological diagnosis. Second, a knowledge of someone's cognitive abilities will allow one to communicate at an appropriate level. Third, the impression given by simple social conversation may be .very misleading. Not infrequently patients who give the appearance of being intellectually challenged are in fact rather sharp and conversely patients with quite serious cognitive impairments can often maintain a social gloss.

Whatever system is used for assessing cognitive functions it should assess orientation, memory, abstract thought and language. When introducing this part of the examination it is wise to warn the patients with something like, 'I am going to do a neurological examination and it starts with asking some questions to see how well your brain is working'. This warns

General physical examination

Temperature	Heart sounds
Blood pressure	Carotid bruits
Pulse	

Higher mental functions

1. *Level of arousal (GCS)*
   a. *Awake and alert*
   b. *Drowsy*
   c. *Stuporous*
   d. *Comatose*
2. Orientation
   a. Person
   b. Place
   c. Date
3. *Commands*
   a. *One-step midline*
   b. *One-step limb*
   c. *Two step*
   d. *Three step*
   e. *Crossing the midline*
4. Memory; 3 objects – immediate recall
5. Cognitive functioning
   a. WORLD
   b. *Proverb*
   c. *Digit span*
   d. Simple maths
6. Language
   a. Naming
   b. Repetition
   c. *Free speech*
7. Memory; 3 objects – recall at 3 minutes

Cranial nerves

I – rarely tested, subjective assessment		
II	a. Fields	
	b. Acuity	
	c. Fundi	
III, IV, VI	a. Movements (nystagmus)	
	b. Diplopia	
	c. PERLA	
V	a. Sensation (LT, PP, cold)	
	b. *Masseter*	
	c. *Corneals (only if appropriate)*	
VII	a. Brow	
	b. Eyes	
	c. Mouth (voluntary and *mimetic*)	
VIII	a. Noise in each ear	
	b. *Rinne*	
	c. *Weber*	
IX, X	a. Palatial movement	
	b. *Quality of speech*	
		i. *Nasal*
		ii. *Guttural*
		iii. *'eee'*
XI	a. Sternoclidomastoid	
	b. *Trapezius*	
XII	a. Tongue movements to command	
	b. *'La' and 'Ta'*	

Limbs

Drift
a. *Bulk (fasciculations)*
b. Tone
c. Power   1/5 = flicker
            2/5 = movement with gravity removed
            3/5 = movement against gravity
            4/5 = against resistance (− and +)
            5/5 = normal
d. Sensation (LT, PP, Cold, Vib, JPS)
e. Co-ordination (FNF, RSM, *RAM, H/S*)

Reflexes

a. *Jaw*	f. *Abdomen*	−/+ = trace or with reinforcement
b. Biceps	g. Knee	+ = present
c. Triceps	h. Ankle	++ = obviously present
d. Supinator	i. Plantars	+++ = pathologically brisk
e. *Finger jerks*		++++ = clonus

Gait

a. Romberg
b. Normal gait (arm swing, width of base)
c. Tandem (forwards, backwards with eyes closed)

Table A1.1 The neurological examination (parts in italics optional)

the patient what is going on and makes it less threatening than launching into questions like, 'Where are you?'. The system I use as a screening test is given in Table A1.1. The details are not important but it is important to have a well-rehearsed system. Level of arousal will usually be obvious, but if abnormal should be recorded in English or using the Glasgow Coma Scale (see Fig. 14.5). Orientation needs to be assessed. The vast majority of patients will get the date correct within a day or two. If they know their location and the date there is no need to ask who they are.

As the neurological examination is full of commands I only do formal commands if the patient is suspected of having an aphasia, or I am having difficulty getting them to do what I want. A one-step midline command would be, 'Close your eyes'. One-step limb would be, 'Show me your thumb'. A two-step command would be, 'Point to the ceiling then point to the floor'. 'Take a piece of paper, fold it in two and place it on the floor' is a three-step command. 'Touch your right ear with your left thumb' is the usual command for crossing the midline. The commands are in order of increasing complexity.

As a screening test I ask patients to remember three objects which are Winston Churchill, Birmingham and a shoe. The objects have to be from different categories and not easily put into a single image. I ask the patient to repeat the three objects and warn them that I shall ask them again in a few minutes. I then ask the patient to spell 'world' forwards and backwards, which despite protestations most patients can do. This is dependent on their educational skills and I use 'hand' or 'cat' if their spelling is not too good. I then ask how many 10 pences there are in £1.50. Again with encouragement most patients can do this. Many doctors ask patients to subtract 7s from 100. I find this test of limited value as many patients cannot do it and find it very stressful.

As a simple assessment of language I ask the patient to name four objects on myself. If there is a suggestion of a problem then I will do further naming with low frequency words, such as lapel or cuff. I ask the patient to repeat the words, 'No ifs, ands or buts about it'. I have already assessed free speech whilst taking the history. Finally I ask what the three objects were I asked them to remember. Adolescents remember all three, while adults remember two to three of the objects. Unless the patient is very nervous remembering one or none out of three is evidence of a memory impairment.

Cranial nerves

I

Cranial nerve I is rarely tested formally with smell bottles, but should be after head trauma or if a frontal lesion is suspected. Anosmia not infrequently occurs after head trauma because the little nerveletts get sheared off as they pass through the cribriform plate. This can obviously have medicolegal consequences so should be documented.

II

Cranial nerve II is the major source of our sensory input. At a minimum three aspects have to be assessed, acuity, fields and the fundoscopic appearance. Although an estimation of acuity can be obtained by reading fine print it is much better to use a Snellen chart and have a reproducible number to compare with. Fields can be done in a number of ways. Examiners tend to feel more comfortable with the wiggly finger method of confrontation. To do this the patient covers an eye and the clinician closes the eye opposite. The clinician then brings a wiggly finger from the periphery theoretically comparing their fields with the patient's. However, for gross movement one's arms are not long enough. All four quadrants should be checked, i.e. 1.30, 4.30, 5.30 and 7.30 using a clock face. For a brief screening test of fields I get the patients to count fingers at the edge of each field in each eye in all four quadrants. If you have an unusually co-operative patient and the patience of Job you can use red matches to plot the red colour fields including the blind spots.

Fundoscopy takes practice. However, it helps if the ophthalmoscope works and is set up correctly, the patient is in a darkened room and is looking at a distant target. Of primary interest to the neurologist is whether the disc is distinct, the absence of papilloedema and the colour of the disc. Venous pulsations, which are evidence of normal intracranial pressure, are difficult to see and should not be relied on.

III, IV, VI

Patients cannot keep their head still while assessing eye movements, so it is necessary to gently lay a hand on the head. A target, such as the end of an expensive pen, makes it more likely the patient will follow the full eye movements. The eyes should be made to fully adduct, abduct, elevate and depress. On lateral gaze it is worth pausing for a few seconds to look for sustained nystagmus. Rapid lateral eye movements may demonstrate a subtle internuclear ophthalmoplegia (see Chapter 10), which may be evidence of MS. The patient should be specifically asked if they experienced double vision. Sometimes what is meant by double vision has to be explained. While looking at the eye movements it is worth pausing to think if there is any ptosis present. Most patients' faces are asymmetrical and it can be tricky deciding if ptosis is present. The relationship between the upper lid and the pupil is the key. If it is different between the two sides then unilateral ptosis is likely to be present. If more than two-fifths of the pupil is covered it is clearly non-functional and may be evidence of bilateral ptosis.

The analysis of a patient complaining of diplopia is relatively simple. Either the diplopia is analysable in terms of single cranial nerves, or it is not. If it is then it will be either a IIIrd nerve palsy or a VIth. An isolated IVth nerve palsy is as rare as the proverbial rocking horse excrement, so is not worth considering. IIIrd nerve palsy will have an associated ptosis and probably dilatation of the pupil. In addition, the images will be at an angle to each other. In a VIth nerve palsy the images are horizontally displaced. There is a failure of full abduction of the eye. When deciding which eye is the source of the diplopia the cover test is useful. The patient looks in the direction in which the diplopia is worst. The fact that there are two images, one of which is further out than the other, is drawn to the patient's attention. An eye is covered and an image will disappear. If the image is from the weak eye then it will be the most displaced, the furthest image. If the diplopia is unanalysable in terms of cranial nerves it could be either brain stem, multiple cranial nerves, a structural lesion in the orbit, muscle pathology or pharmacological (e.g. carbamazepine toxicity). It is worth looking for fatiguability in diplopia (the diplopia gets worse on keeping the eyes in a displaced position) as it might be evidence of myasthenia gravis.

Less than 1 mm anisocoria (asymmetry of pupil size) is usually of no significance. Pupils can be tested for response to light both directly (shining the light into the eye being tested) and consensually (shining the light in the other eye). The response is greater in a darkened room. Response to accommodation is often difficult to demonstrate, particularly in the elderly. The patient should be asked to look at a distant target and then asked to focus on a near target. I often ask them to read the time from my watch, held about 15 cm from their nose.

V

When testing the Vth (trigeminal) cranial nerve, it is worth remembering it is made up of three divisions, ophthalmic, maxillary and mandibular. Sensation should be tested in all three and compared with the opposite side. Routinely I only test pin prick, but light touch and temperature can easily be done. The corneal reflexes are not done routinely, but are mandatory if a trigeminal nerve problem is suspected. They are performed by touching the cornea with a twisted piece of tissue. Both the objective reaction and the subjective sensation should be assessed.

VII

Although the VIIth (facial) nerve is not organized into three divisions, it is useful to test it as if it were. Movements of the brow, round the eyes, and mouth should be assessed. If there is a weakness then consideration should be given as to whether it is of an upper motor neurone or lower motor neurone pattern. If the damage is to the facial nerve itself (lower motor neurone) then the whole of the face on that side is likely to be affected. If the damage is at a cortical or white track level (upper motor neurone), as there is bilateral representation of the upper face at an upper motor neurone level, it takes bilateral damage to cause brow weakness. So the usual pattern of weakness in a unilateral upper motor neurone lesion affecting the face is of weakness around the mouth, less around the eye and none of the brow. Fortunately God gave us two sides of the body so neurologists could compare them. However, this does mean that bilateral facial weakness can be missed. Ptosis is not a sign of facial (VII) weakness.

VIII

Some assessment of the VIIIth nerve should be made on all patients. This may only be by checking that the rubbing of two fingers can be heard equally loudly in each ear. Unilateral deafness should not be dismissed as it may be the only evidence of an acoustic neuroma. The Weber and Rinne tests can be performed to further type any hearing loss. The Rinne test consists of asking the patient to compare the loudness of sound transmitted through air, by placing a tuning fork close to the external auditory meatus, or through bone, by placing the base of the tuning fork against the mastoid bone behind the ear. Usually air conduction is better than bone. In conductive deafness (where there is a problem of transmission of the noise from the external auditor meatus to the cochlea) bone conduction is better than air, as it avoids the area where there is a problem. In profound sensory neural deafness (where there is a problem in the cochlea or auditory nerve) sometimes bone conduction appears louder than air if the noise is being transmitted through the skull to the functioning ear. In the Weber test the base of the tuning fork is placed in the middle of the forehead at the hair line and the patient has to say whether the noise is loudest in the middle or at either ear. Normally it is louder in the centre. In sensory neural deafness it is heard louder towards the good ear. Paradoxically in conducive deafness it is heard loudest towards the deaf ear. One can test this on oneself by sticking a finger in an external auditor meatus and performing the Weber test on oneself.

IX, X

By listening to the patient and discerning that there is no dysarthria one has already started the assessment of the IXth and Xth cranial nerves. If it is necessary to assess the Xth further then the patient can be asked to make a high-pitched 'eee' sound, as this requires the adduction of the vocal cords. Getting the patient to open their mouth to see the palate rise symmetrically is all that is required on routine clinical examination. The gag reflex is usually done for the wrong reason in that it is an inadequate assessment of swallowing. The only time it is of much use is when a patient has a bulbar palsy and it is necessary to differentiate bulbar from pseudo-bulbar. When it is necessary to assess swallowing the best test is to see what happens when the patient attempts to swallow a small amount of water. In neurogenic causes of dysphagia liquids are much more difficult than solids. If the patient coughs after swallowing then some aspiration is occurring. A more subtle test of swallowing is a timed test of swallowing 150 ml of water. Most people under 75 can swallow 10 ml per second.

XI

I do not test the XIth nerve routinely.

XII

When the patient has opened their mouth the tongue's bulk can be noted. Looking for fasciculations in the tongue is extremely tricky as patients have a problem in relaxing their tongues (in common with a number of people I know). As a routine I ask patients to rapidly move their tongue from side to side after sticking it out. There is a wide variation in normal for this capacity.

Limbs

Some deeply irritating people refer to the limbs as the peripheral nervous system (PNS). This is incorrect as both the CNS and PNS are being assessed when the limbs are examined. In each limb an assessment of tone, power, sensation and co-ordination should be made. The first step is ask the patient to hold their hands out with the palms uppermost and the eyes closed. Drift can be either due to motor or proprioceptive dysfunction. The bulk of muscles should be observed, particularly the small muscles of the hands. In the appropriate circumstances fasciculations should be looked for. This requires some time, adequate exposure and the muscles being relaxed. Tone in the upper extremities should be assessed at the elbow and wrist. In the lower extremities if the patient is lying down and relaxed when the knee is suddenly lifted the ankle remains on the couch. However, many patients are not relaxed enough for this to work. Tone should be assessed at the knee and the ankle forcibly dorsiflexed with the knee flexed for the elicitation of clonus. Pain makes the assessment of tone impossible.

Power should be assessed across the shoulder, elbow, wrist,. finger, hip, knee, and ankle joints. It is recorded with the MRC grading system (Table A1.1), but is often better expressed in English, for example 'there was mild proximal weakness in the lower extremities'. The MRC scale has to be adjusted to the patient's general condition. Statements such that the patient was 4+/5 throughout the body is a nonsense.

A screening examination of sensation should go distally in each limb, as the most likely abnormality to be picked up is a peripheral neuropathy. If the context dictates a much more thorough examination may be appropriate, but testing of light touch, pin prick, cold, vibration and joint position sense in the fingers and toes is usually more than adequate. It is more subtle and revealing not to ask the patients whether or not these modalities are perceived, but whether their perception is normal and similar to that in other parts of the body.

To test co-ordination I routinely test foot tap, rapidly touching the thumb with the fingers, and the finger-nose-finger test. Rapid alternating movements and the heal shin test are useful additions when appropriate.

Reflexes

Any muscle with two attachments can demonstrate a deep tendon reflex, but the traditional and easiest elicitable are the biceps, supinator, triceps, knee and ankle. The tendon has to be put under tension and a brief sharp tap with the hammer will produce a responding jerk. Anxious people have brisk reflexes which can cause some confusion. Absence of deep tendon reflexes is always pathological. The jaw jerk is useful when there is hyper-reflexia in all four limbs. If the jaw jerk is not pathological then a high cervical myelopathy is the most likely cause, whereas if the jaw jerk is brisk then the pathology extends above the foramen magnum. The abdominal reflexes are superficial cutaneous reflexes and are lost in CNS pathology, so the presence of abdominal reflexes in the presence of bilateral leg weakness would be against a myelopathy. The plantar reflex is a response to a noxious stimulus to the sole of the foot performed to look for a Babinski or extensor reaction. The Babinski response is a phylogenetically older response than the normal pyramidal response which is toe flexion. It is evidence of pathology in the pyramidal tract from the cortex down.

Gait

What often differentiates the examination performed by a neurologist from the non-neurologist is that the neurologist will attempt to walk the patient. The patient may not be able to walk, but how that most basic of functions fails often gives valuable insight into the pathological process. For example, truncal ataxia may not be apparent until the patient sits on the edge of the bed attempting to stand. Some gaits are classical. Wide-based gaits suggest cerebellar pathology. A stamping gait is said to be typical of tabes dorsalis, but is seen in any condition where proprioception is impaired. The festinating, stooped gait of Parkinson's disease is often diagnostic.

The Romberg test is traditionally supposed to test proprioception. The patient stands with the eyes closed. The three systems that tell someone where they are in space are the vestibular system, visual input and proprioception. If vision is taken out by closing the eyes and proprioception is lost then the vestibular system is insufficient to keep the patient upright.

BP 140/80, HS I & II & 0 No carotid bruits

HMF, O × 3, naming, repetition, $\overset{\longrightarrow}{\underset{\longleftarrow}{WORLD}}$, 1.50 = 15, remembers 3/3 at 3 minutes

CNs IÖ, II Fields full, fundi OK acuity 6/6 bilaterally
III, IV, VI, full, PERLA
V✓, VII✓, VIII✓, IX X✓, XII✓

Arms and legs, no drift
Tone, power and sensation to LT, PP, cold, vib and JPS normal
FNF, and RSM normal

DTR	B	T	S	K	A	P
R	+	+	+	+	+	↓
L	+	+	+	+	+	↓

Gait – normal. Tandem OK, Romberg −ve

Table A1.2 The neurological examination recorded

The tandem gait (heel to toe) is a good test of cerebellar function. Patients under 60 can do it backwards with the eyes closed. It is important to be close enough to catch the patient if they fall.

The neurological examination gives a lot of information about the patient. Done slickly it can be a tour de force and great fun both for the examiner and patient. It is important that it is adequately recorded (Table A1.2) as changes from day to day, week to week or year to year may be important.

Appendix 2 – How to do a lumbar puncture

Like the neurological examination lumbar puncture (LP) is a skilled motor activity at which one only gets proficient with practice. It also requires at least a degree of co-operation from the patient and so gaining and keeping the patient's trust is vital. Usually it is a straightforward and virtually painless procedure taking about half an hour. However, it can be traumatic for both patient and lumbar-puncturist, so before embarking on it ask yourself, 'Is this procedure necessary?'. Circumstances where it is mandatory are suspicion of subarachnoid haemorrhage after a negative CT and suspicion of meningitis in a relatively well patient, also after a negative CT. Once you have decided it is necessary you have committed yourself to a course of action of doing whatever is necessary to obtain CSF. It would be difficult to defend the position of at one stage thinking an LP was necessary, but when it became technically difficult abandoning the procedure.

Contraindications

If there is a potential for herniation one should not be doing an LP. Causes of herniation are non-communicating hydrocephalus, mass lesions and cerebral oedema. The vast majority of patients will have had an imaging study of the brain prior to an LP to exclude these possibilities. One should never be dependent on the presence or absence of papilloedema to determine if an LP should be performed. It is a late and unreliable sign of raised intracranial pressure and may not be a contraindication to lumbar puncture, e.g. communicating hydrocephalus or benign intracranial hypertension. Bleeding diathesis, such as a prolonged prothrombin time or low platelets, increase the risk of an epidural haematoma and are relative contraindications. Previous surgery to the lum-

bar spine will make a lumbar puncture more difficult and increase the likelihood of low back pain following the procedure. Arachnoiditis and anatomical abnormalities such as tethered cord will significantly add to the risks of the procedure.

Preparing the patient

The first step is to talk to the patient. Explain why you want to do an LP and what you will be doing. I tell the patients that I want them to tell me exactly what they are feeling and I shall tell them what I am doing. While one is talking to the patient one can make some assessment of their anxiety level. Patients have often heard about the horrors of 'lumbar punch' and may have had a previous adverse experience. While reassurance will overcome some of this anxiety 10 mg of diazepam orally an hour before the procedure, or a reasonable dose of opiates, will relieve anxiety and help the lumbar paraspinal musculature to relax, so facilitating the procedure.

The lateral position

The majority of patients will have their LP performed in the lateral position, a few will need to sit up.

The patient is laid on their side with a pillow supporting their head and their knees drawn up in a 'fetal' position. The patient lies at the edge of the bed and the idea is to get the spine as straight as possible (Table A2.1). While the LP can be performed by a single operative without assistance it is a kindness to have a nurse on the other side of the bed holding the patient's hand.

There is more than one way to skin a rabbit and the procedure I describe is the one I have

Is it necessary?
Are there contraindications?
   Mass in the head
   Non-communicating
   Hydrocephalus
   Bleeding diathesis
Inform patient
Position patient
Identify landmarks
Insert local anaesthetic
Set up trolley
Insert LP needle
Measure opening pressure
Collect CSF
Withdraw LP needle and clean up patient
Draw bloods
Label and send off samples
Clean up trolley including sharps
Record LP in the notes
Go back and check patient is OK

Table A2.1 Steps in performing an LP

the spinous processes and draw a line along them which gives me the midline. I choose a gap between the processes that is easily palpated below my L3 line and mark this with a small box. As my drawing may well be washed off by the antiseptic I draw radiating lines to point me to the space I have identified (Fig. A2.1). After the use of an alcohol swab, using a fine needle I introduce a bleb of 2% lignocaine intradermally. Once the skin is numb using a green needle (21 gauge) I introduce about 1–2 ml of lignocaine along the track I shall use for the LP needle. The green needle is too short to reach the dura, but I aspirate prior to injecting more local to make sure I am not in a blood vessel. With the green needle I have explored the initial path of my LP needle and made sure that I will avoid a spinous process. While the local anaesthetic is working I then set up my LP trolley with some gauze swabs, a little pot of antiseptic, a manometer, and an LP needle. There is evidence that bevelled needles produce less in the way of low pressure headache, but they are more expensive so usually not available. The greater the bore of the needle the stiffer it is and the easier it is to do the LP. However, the finer the needle the less likely will be a post LP headache. The standard

found effective, but others will use slightly different techniques. Having put the patient in the correct position I place my index fingers on the top of the iliac crests (hips) and have my thumbs meeting in the midline. I then draw a line across the back at this level which is approximately L3. If I do not go above this level I shall not hit the conus. I then palpate

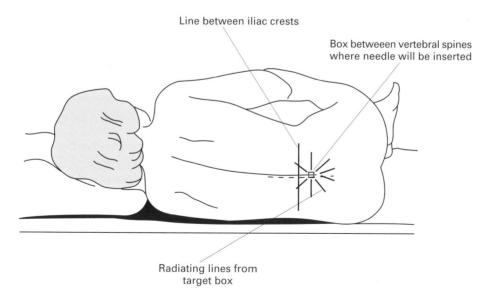

Line between iliac crests

Box betweeen vertebral spines
where needle will be inserted

Radiating lines from
target box

Fig. A2.1 The lateral position for performing a lumbar puncture, with marks to guide where to put the needle.

needle is a 20 gauge. I place a green drape under the patient's back covering the bed below the LP site to stop CSF and blood staining the sheets. I do not fully drape the LP site as these drapes are of only cosmetic utility and often get in the way. Once I have set up my trolley I put on sterile gloves and using the gauze and antiseptic clean the site of the LP and a wide area of skin around it. When using iodine it is a good idea to check with the patient they are not allergic to it prior to its application. I clean the actual LP site a second time. I am now ready to insert the needle.

Inserting the needle

I warn the patient of what I am about to do and tell them to curl in a little ball, but ensuring their shoulders remain vertical. The needle should be inserted pointing slightly caudally. It should be done with a good idea of where the midline is. There is a fair amount of resistance as one goes through muscle and ligaments. Bones bring the needle to a firm halt and often pain for the patient as the periostium is pain sensitive. There is a final resistance before entering the subarachnoid space. Often the patient experiences a pain in the back at this point. If you prang a nerve root the patient feels an electric feeling going down the leg. This will go on repositioning the needle. The subarachnoid space is usually deeper than you think, between 5 and 10 cm. In obese people the LP needle may well be in up to the hilt before you hit CSF. Occasionally a standard needle will not be long enough. Once you think you are in remove the stilette and after a couple of seconds a clear fluid will hopefully emerge. Attach the manometer to the needle and measure the pressure. It would be helpful to have as many hands as Brahma at this point, but with practice two will suffice. If the patient gives a small cough the pressure should rise and fall. Remove the manometer and fill your bottles with CSF, not forgetting the glucose bottle. Between 10 and 15 drops per bottle is sufficient. If you are doing the LP

to look for malignant cells the more CSF taken the more likely they are to be found. Many people get an assistant to hold the bottles under the needle. As I am not going to be introducing anything into the patient from this stage on I allow myself to be de-sterilized and pick up the bottles myself. Whoever holds the bottles should be wearing gloves as CSF is a body fluid and potentially infectious. Once sufficient CSF is obtained the needle is pulled out, the site cleaned up and a small plaster placed over the hole. The patient is advised to lie flat for a couple of hours.

Sitting up position

This is an easier approach as the midline is not obscured by slabs of adipose tissue hanging over the spinal processes. However, it makes it much more difficult to estimate the opening pressure. The patient is sat with their back at the edge of the bed hunched over an adjustable table with a couple of pillows on it. The procedure is the same as in the lateral position, except that once the needle is in and a few drops of CSF have been seen the stilette is replaced. If the opening pressure is important then the patient is then rotated into a lateral position. This is tricky and requires two people, one to take care of the LP needle and one to help the patient lie on their side in a controlled fashion. Even so, the needle can become displaced, so if the opening pressure is not important it is easier to get the CSF out in the sitting position. Once the patient is in a lying position one waits a minute or so before measuring the pressure with the manometer.

Handling samples and recording in the notes

After finishing the LP care must be taken of the precious samples. Blood will also need to be drawn if paired glucose readings are needed or for oligoclonal bands. The samples need to be clearly labelled and the appropriate forms filled in. Transport of the samples to the laboratory should be arranged. The thought of having to repeat an LP because a sample is 'lost' is not an appealing one. In some hospitals where I have worked such was the reliability of the portering system and the laboratories that I kept a spare sample of CSF in the refrigerator until results were available.

In the notes record the date and time of the procedure and what samples were taken and what they were sent for. Clear up your own LP trolley. You are responsible for your own sharps and an LP trolley is likely to be a mess after use. It is unfair and unprofessional to expect nursing staff to clear up after our mess, particularly if dangerous sharps are present.

After care of the patient

The patient should lie flat for at least 2 hours. They may need minor analgesics for back pain. A good proportion of patients develop a low pressure headache. This can be very unpleasant with pain, nausea and neck stiffness. It goes if the patient lies flat. It is due to a persistent leak of CSF from the hole made in the dura. Usually it is self-limiting and goes within 24 hours. Sometimes it is persistent and can be cured with a blood patch. This consists of injecting 10 ml of the patient's own blood into the area of the hole in the dura. It is quite a tricky procedure and best undertaken by people experienced in it.

What to do when you can't get in

Stop. With repeated failed attempts at passing the needle both operator and patient soon get stressed out. Before you have entirely used all the patient's good will, stop. Clean the patient up. Go away and have a cup of coffee. If there is a colleague available get them to try as often a fresh pair of hands will do the LP with sickening alacrity. The patient may well benefit from 10 mg of diazepam pretreatment. If a couple of people have failed then the LP should be performed under X-ray guidance.

Appendix 3 – Final MCQs and answers to MCQs

Chapter 1	Chapter 2	Chapter 3	Chapter 4	Chapter 5
1. FTTF	1. TFTF	1. TFFT	1. FTFT	1. FTFT
2. TFTF	2. TFTF	2. TTFF	2. FTTF	2. FFTT
3. FFFT	3. FFTT	3. FFTT	3. TTFF	3. TTFF
4. TFFT	4. TTFT	4. TTTF	4. TTFF	4. FFTT
5. TFFT	5. FFTF	5. FTTF	5. TFFT	5. TFTF
6. TTTF	6. TFTF	6. TTTT	6. FTTF	6. TFFT
7. FTFT	7. TTFT	7. FTTF	7. FTTT	7. FFTT
8. TTFF	8. TFTF	8. TFFT	8. TFFT	8. TFTF
9. TTFF	9. FTTF	9. FTFT	9. FFTT	9. TFFT
10. TTFT	10. TTTF	10. FFTT	10. TFTT	10. TTFF

Chapter 6	Chapter 7	Chapter 8	Chapter 9	Chapter 10
1. TTFF	1. TTFT	1. FTTF	1. FFTT	1. FTTF
2. TFTF	2. TFFF	2. TTFF	2. TTFF	2. FTTT
3. TTFF	3. TTFF	3. FFFF	3. FTFT	3. FFTT
4. TFFT	4. TFTF	4. TTFF	4. FFTT	4. FTFF
5. FFTT	5. FFTT	5. FFTT	5. TTFF	5. FTTF
6. FTTT	6. TTFT	6. FTFF	6. FTFT	6. FTFT
7. FTFT	7. TFTF	7. TTFT	7. TTFF	7. TTFF
8. FTTF	8. TTFF	8. FFTT	8. FTTF	8. FTFT
9. TTFF	9. FFFT	9. FTTT	9. TFFT	9. TTTF
10. TFFT	10. TTFF	10. FTFF	10. TTFF	10. FFFT

Chapter 11	Chapter 12	Chapter 13	Chapter 14	Chapter 15
1. TFTF	1. FTTF	1. FTTF	1. TFTF	1. TTFF
2. FFTT	2. FFTT	2. FFTT	2. FTFT	2. TTFF
3. TFTF	3. FFTT	3. TTFF	3. TTFF	3. FFTT
4. FTTF	4. FFFT	4. TFTF	4. TFTF	4. FTFT
5. FTTF	5. TTTF	5. FTTF	5. TTTF	5. TFTF
6. FTTF	6. TTFT	6. FTFT	6. FTFF	6. TFTF
7. TTFF	7. TFTF	7. TFTF	7. TTFF	7. FTTF
8. TTFT	8. TFFT	8. TFTF	8. TFTF	8. TTFF
9. FFFT	9. TFTT	9. TFFT	9. FTTF	9. TTFF
10. FTFT	10. FTTT	10. TFTF	10. TFTF	10. TTTT

Chapter 16	Chapter 17	Chapter 18	Chapter 19	Chapter 20
1. TTFF	1. TFFT	1. TTFT	1. TTFF	1. TFFT
2. FTTF	2. FTFT	2. TFTT	2. TFTF	2. TFTF
3. TTTF	3. FTTF	3. FFFF	3. FTTT	3. TFFT
4. FTFF	4. TTFT	4. TFFT	4. FFTF	4. TFTF
5. FTFF	5. FFFT	5. TTFF	5. TFTF	5. FTTF
6. FFTT	6. TTTF	6. TFFT	6. FFTT	6. TTFF
7. TTFF	7. FTFT	7. FTTT	7. TTFF	7. TFTF
8. TFTT	8. FFTT	8. FFFT	8. FFTT	8. FTFT
9. TTFF	9. FFTT	9. FFTT	9. TTFF	9. FFTT
10. FTFT	10. TTFF	10. TTFF	10. TTTT	10. TTFF

Final MCQs

The MCQs are either true T or false F. The answers are given at the end of this appendix. Negatively mark your answers; a point for a correct answer, deduct a point for an incorrect response. If you score 40 or more you pass.

1. **Neuroanatomy:**
   A The central sulcus divides the frontal from the temporal lobe.
   B Broca's area is in the parietal lobe.
   C The primary auditory area is in the temporal lobe.
   D The frontal lobes are important for planning.

2.
   A The dermatomal supply for the umbilicus is T10.
   B The biceps jerk is C5/6.
   C The ulnar nerve can get compressed in the carpal tunnel.
   D The common peroneal nerve supplies muscles involved in plantar flexion.

3. **Features of upper motor neurone lesions include:**
   A Fasciculations.
   B Hyper-reflexia.
   C Primitive reflexes.
   D Hypotonia.

4. **Brain-stem signs include:**
   A Crossed motor and sensory syndromes.
   B Nystagmus.
   C Aphasia.
   D Homonimous hemianopsia.

5.
   A Conduction is slowed in axonal neuropathies.
   B The direction of nystagmus is given by the slow phase.
   C The medial longitudinal fasciculus connects the VIth and IIIrd nerve nuclei.
   D The EEG can be diagnostically useful in herpes encephalitis.

6. **The headache of raised intracranial pressure is classically:**
   A Worse in the mornings.
   B Relieved by coughing.
   C Unilateral.
   D May be complicated by visual obscurations.

7. **In the Brown–Séquard syndrome:**
   A Weakness is ipsilateral to the lesion.
   B Spinothalamic loss is contralateral to the lesion.
   C Joint position sense loss is contralateral to the lesion.
   D An extensor plantar response is usually contralateral.

8. **Causes of intrinsic cord pathology include:**
   A HIV.
   B Meningioma.
   C B_{12} deficiency.
   D Hydrocephalus.

9. **Causes of mononeuritis multiplex include:**
   A Thyrotoxicosis.
   B Rheumatoid disease.
   C Diabetes mellitus.
   D Lead poisoning.

10.
   A Duchenne muscular dystrophy is more common in girls than boys.
   B Dystrophia myotonica is autosomal recessive.
   C Inclusion-body myositis responds to steroids.
   D Mitochondrial DNA is inherited from the mother.

11.
   A Trigeminal neuralgia responds well to carbamazepine.
   B Epileptic seizures are always preceded by an aura.
   C Lhermitte's sign is suggestive of cervical cord demyelination.
   D Fatigue is a common symptom of MS.

12. Cerebrovascular disease:
  A TIAs can last up to 48 hours.
  B Temporal arteritis rarely occurs in patients under 50 years of age.
  C Hypertensive haemorrhages are frequently lobar.
  D Venous sinus thrombosis can complicate pregnancy.

13. Epilepsy:
  A The prevalence of epilepsy is about 1%.
  B Primary generalized epilepsy may be preceded by *déjà vu.*
  C Phenytoin can cause coarsening of facial features.
  D Carbamazepine is not teratogenic.

14. Multiple sclerosis:
  A The incidence in Northern Europeans is 1/800.
  B Internuclear ophthalmoplegia suggests cortical involvement.
  C MRI is the most sensitive investigation.
  D Primary progressive MS is the most common subtype.

15. Parkinson's disease:
  A Can be caused by carbon monoxide poisoning.
  B Often responds to Sinemet.
  C Pergolide is a dopamine agonist.
  D Hallucinations may complicate treatment.

16.
  A Juvenile myoclonic epilepsy usually responds to valproate.
  B Narcolepsy is associated with HLA DW4.
  C Wilson's disease is a disorder of iron metabolism.
  D Motor neurone disease does not have upper motor neurone signs.

17.
  A Status epilepticus should be broken within 1 hour.
  B Non-epileptic seizure disorder can present as status.
  C A CT of the head will usually diagnose the cause of coma.
  D A Glasgow Coma Scale score of $0 =$ death.

18. In the neurological examination:
  A Rapid lateral eye movements may reveal an internuclear ophthalmoplegia.
  B VIth nerve palsies are associated with ptosis.
  C Ptosis is a sign of a VIIth nerve palsy.
  D Abdominal reflexes are brisk in cord compression.

19. Brain tumours:
  A Acoustic neuromas arise on the acoustic nerve.
  B Pituitary adenomas can present with bitemporal field deficits.
  C Glioblastoma multiforme has a bad prognosis.
  D Median survival with cerebral metastases is 18 weeks.

20. Encephalopathies:
  A Creutzfeld–Jakob disease is caused by prions.
  B A construction apraxia is common in hepatic encephalopathy.
  C Hypertensive encephalopathy is rarely associated with papilloedema.
  D Ethanol rarely causes a toxic encephalopathy.

Answers to final MCQs

1. FFTT	2. TTFF	3. FTTF
4. TTFF	5. FFTT	6. TFFT
7. TTFF	8. TFTF	9. FTTF
10. FFFT	11. TFTT	12. FTFT
13. TFTF	14. TFTF	15. FTTT
16. TFFF	17. TTFF	18. TFFF
19. FTTT	20. TTFF	

Appendix 4 – Glossary

abscess localized area of infection with a liquefied centre and surrounding wall

abduction away from the body

acoustic neuroma misnamed Schwannoma, usually of the vestibular nerve

acromegally disease due to excessive growth hormone from the pituitary

acyclovir drug with anti-herpes activity

adduction movement towards the body

afferents fibres going into the CNS

akinesia slowness or lack of movement

albinism autosomal condition, lacking melanin pigmentation with blond hair, pale skin and pink eyes

Alzheimer's disease commonest form of dementia

amaurosis fugax a TIA in the eye causing transient visual loss

amenorrhoea loss of periods

amitriptyline in low dose used for headache and other neurological pain syndromes, in high dose an antidepressant

amygdala a nucleus in the temporal lobe which is involved in memory and emotion

amyloid protein resistant to degradation made into a beta pleated sheet

amyotrophy muscle atrophy

angiography imaging the blood vessels

angor animi fear of imminent doom

anhydrosis absence of sweat

anisocoria unequal pupils

anosmia loss of sense of smell

anoxia lack of oxygen

anterior at the front

antiemetic medication for treating nausea and vomiting

aperient laxative

aphasia difficulty with language. The same as dysphasia, the latter being used more in the UK

apraxia the lack of the knowledge about how to do something

aqueduct of Sylvius small tube through which CSF flows from the IIIrd to the IVth ventricle

arachnoid villi area where CSF is reabsorbed into the sagittal sinus

arachnoiditis chronic scarring inflammation of the arachnoid

arcuate fasciculus white matter tract that links Wernicke's and Broca's areas

areflexia absent deep tendon reflexes

arrhythmogenic has the propensity to produce cardiac arrhythmias

arteriovenous malformation abnormal collection of blood vessels

arteritis inflammation of arteries

aspiration pneumonia pneumonia due to the inhalation of food or secretions. A common complication of bulbar muscular inco-ordination

astrocytoma form of glioma derived from astrocytes

ataxia unsteadiness; often seen in cerebellar disease

atheroma collection of cholesterol, lipid and inflammatory cells that forms on the inside of blood vessels

atherosclerosis narrowing in arteries due to atheroma – complex combination of lipids, complex carbohydrates, blood products and fibrous tissue

atropine anticholinergic (muscarinic)

Babinski phenomena extension of the great toe with fanning of the toes on application of a noxious stimulus to the outer sole

Behçet's disease rare vasculitis

benzodiazepines group of sedative drugs

Binswanger's encephalopathy multi-infarct dementia due to white matter ischaemia

bitemporal field loss visual loss in both temporal fields associated with pituitary tumours

bradycardia slow heart rate

Broca's area area at the lower end of the motor strip in the posterior frontal lobe responsible for the articulation and syntax of speech

bromocriptine dopamine agonist

Brown–Séquard syndrome constellation of signs seen in hemisection of the cord

bulbar palsy weakness of the muscles supplied by the cranial nerves that come from the bulb area of the brain stem, i.e. swallowing and articulation

caeruloplasmin protein in blood for carrying copper

carbamazepine an anti-epileptic drug

cardioplegia stopped heart

carpal tunnel tunnel at the wrist through which the median nerve passes

carpal tunnel syndrome entrapment of the median nerve at the wrist

cauda equina the nerve roots that stream down from the conus (Latin for horse's tail)

caudal towards the tail (downwards)

caudate a nucleus in the basal ganglia

causalgia pain syndrome where normal sensations are interpreted as painful

cerebrospinal fluid (CSF) the fluid bathing the brain and spinal cord

cerebrovascular pertaining to the blood vessels that supply the brain

cervical spondylosis degenerative disease of the cervical cord

chemotaxis attracting cells by chemical messages

Chiari malformation congenital malformation whose cardinal feature is displacement of the cerebellar tonsils through the foramen magnum

chiasma cross over; particularly where the optic nerves meet

chorea irregular twisting and writhing movements

choreiform resembles chorea

choreoathetosis chorea with a writhing component

choroid plexus area where CSF is made

circle of Willis circular arrangement of the blood vessels at the base of the brain

cirrhosis scarring of the liver

claudication pain on exercise secondary to ischaemia

colliculi two small hills at the back of the mesencephalon involved in vision and hearing

computerized axial tomography (CT) the technique of shining X-rays through a structure in 365° and using the resulting loss of X-ray energy due to absorption to build up a two-dimensional image

conductive hearing loss deafness due to dysfunction before the cochlea, the commonest being wax in the ear

consensually with respect to the light reflex, the response seen in the eye opposite to the one with the light shining in it

contractures shortening of tendons

contralateral the other side

contrast dye used to enhance images, either X-ray or MRI

conus medullaris also known simply as the conus, the end of the spinal cord

copralalia the uttering of obscenities

corona radiata radiation of white matter tracts from the internal capsule to the cortex

corpus callosum the largest white matter tract linking the two hemispheres

corticosteroids steroids with properties similar to those secreted by the adrenal cortex, their major therapeutic effects are as replacement, anti-inflammatory and as an immunosuppressant

cranial of, or towards, the head

craniopharyngioma embryonic tumour of the pituitary area

craniotomy opening the skull

creatine kinase muscle enzyme

Creutzfeld–Jakob disease (CJD) a spongiform encephalopathy with a new version linked to BSE

cribriform plate bone through which the nerveletts of the first cranial nerve pass

cuneate nucleus nucleus in the brain stem that receives the posterior column sensory input from the arms

Cushing's disease condition where excessive amounts of corticosteroids are made

cytotoxic cell killing

decubitus ulcer ulcer or pressure sore from lying flat

decussate cross over sides

demyelination the pathological process of damage to the myelin sheaths around neurones – seen in MS

dendo-rubro-pallido-luysian atrophy autosomal dominant ataxia

denervation loss of neuronal input, as where nerves die and a muscle is left without nervous attachment

depolarization change in membrane potential in excitable cells

dermatome embryological term for the area of skin that is derived from a segment and takes its sensory supply from a particular nerve root, e.g. the C5 dermatome

dermatomyositis inflammatory myositis with skin involvement

dexamethasone powerful corticosteroid

diabetes insipidus loss of, or loss of response, to AVP resulting in a diuresis

diabetic ketoacidosis (DKA) condition in which large amounts of ketones are in the blood with a high blood sugar due to a lack of insulin

diastolic lowest blood pressure in the cardiac cycle

diplegia both legs paralysed

diplopia double vision

discectomy removal of a disc

disequilibrium unsteadiness

disinhibited loss of the usual social inhibitions

disassociation when neurological findings do not occur together, usually because of the anatomy of the tracts, e.g. Brown–Séquard

dissection (of an artery) a tear in the inner wall with the production of a false lumen and the risk of occlusion or embolization

distal converse of proximal

dopamine neurotransmitter

dorsal back

dorsiflexion pulling the foot back

Duchenne muscular dystrophy X-linked autosomal recessive progressive muscle disease of childhood

dura toughest and most external of the meninges

dysaesthesiae abnormal and usually unpleasant cutaneous sensation

dysarthria failure of articulation

dysphagia difficulties with swallowing

dysphasia difficulty with language. The same as aphasia, the latter being used more in North America

dystaxia ataxia; unsteadiness

dystonia abnormal movements due to failure of control of underlying muscle tone

dystrophies inherited progressive muscle diseases usually presenting in childhood

Edinger–Westphal nucleus nucleus intimate with the IIIrd nerve nuclei responsible for accommodation

efferents fibres coming out of the CNS

embolus a bit of matter foreign to the blood stream that is carried through the blood stream until it gets stuck, e.g. a clot in pulmonary embolism

encephalitis inflammation of the brain, e.g. herpes simplex encephalitis

encephalopathy brain dysfunction, with global connotations

enophthalmos orbit going in

ependyma lining of the ventricular system and central canal of the cord

ependymoma malignant tumour arising from ependymal cells which line the ventricular system and the central canal of the spinal cord

epidural outside the dura, otherwise known as extradural

evulsion ripping off

extension straightening of a joint

extra- outside

extracellular outside the cell

extramedullary outside the spinal cord

FTA Fluorescent treponemal antibody absorbed – specific test for syphilis

fasciculation clinically, the spontaneous twitching of parts of muscles. Physiologically it is the firing of a motor unit, the alpha motor neurone and all the fascicles of muscle attached to it

fasciculus small bundle, as in muscle fascicle or nerve fibre tract

fatiguability decreasing muscular power with time

festinating description of a gait with lots of little rapid steps

festinating gait many small steps – typical in Parkinson's disease

flexion bending of a joint

foramen magnum big hole at the base of the skull where the spinal cord meets the brain

fossa   Latin for a ditch, used for any hollowed out area, e.g. posterior fossa

foviate   bring an image onto the macula

functional   non-organic

gadolinium   metal used as a basis for various contrast agents in MR scanning, the commonest being gadolinium-EDTA

ganglion   a junction box for nerves

gastrocnemius   large muscle in the calf

glabellar tap   on percussing the middle of the forehead subjects will involuntarily blink. Normally this response rapidly fatigues, not so in Parkinsonism

glioblastoma multiforme   most malignant astrocytoma

glioma   commonest form of primary brain tumour derived from glial cells

gliosis   scarring in the brain with glial cells

globus pallidus   a nucleus in the basal ganglia

gracile nucleus   nucleus in the brain stem that receives the posterior column input from the legs

graphaesthesiae   the ability to tactilely perceive complex patterns drawn on the skin

Guillain–Barré syndrome   an acute demyelinating peripheral neuropathy which often follows a viral infection

haematogenous   via the blood stream

Hallpike manoeuvre   moving the patient from the sitting to the lying position while looking for nystagmus or the complaint of vertigo; originally described by Bárány

hemibalismus   violent movements of the limbs

hemiplegia   paralysis of an arm and leg on the same side

hemisection   cut through half

herniate   refers to the movement of the brain from one compartment to another and requires a pressure gradient

herniated nucleus pulposus (HNP)   slipped disc

hippocampus   structure in the medial temporal lobe with a role in memory

histology   examination of tissue under a microscope

homonymous hemianopia (-anopsia)   loss of vision for the same half of the visual world in both eyes

homunculus   literally little man, it refers to the distorted representation of the body in the sensory cortex

humoral   in the blood

hyaline degeneration   changes in small arterioles brought on by hypertension

hydrocephalus   water on the brain

hyper-reflexia   increased deep tendon reflexes

hyperacusis   noises appearing louder than usual

hypercalcaemia   high calcium

hyponatraemia   low sodium

hypoperfusion   reduced perfusion as in cerebral ischaemia

hypophysectomy   removal of the pituitary

hyporeflexia   reduced or absent deep tendon reflexes

hypotension   low blood pressure

hypoxia   lack of oxygen

iatrogenic   caused by doctors

ictus   Latin for a blow; sudden event, e.g. stroke or seizure

idiopathic   cause unknown

incontinence   lack of control, usually of urine or faeces, but can be emotion

infarct   area of dead tissue, usually secondary to ischaemia

inferior   below

inotrop   influencing cardiac muscle activity

internuclear ophthalmoplegia (INO)   failure to co-ordinate the two eyes due to a lesion of the medial longitudinal fasciculus (MLF)

intra-   inside

intracellular   inside the cell

intracerebral   inside the brain

intracranial   inside the cranium, i.e. skull

intradural   inside the dura

intraparenchymal   inside the substance, usually of the brain

intrathecal   inside the theca (sheath); in the subarachnoid space

intravascular compartment   volume inside blood vessels

intubate   insert an endotracheal tube

ipsilateral   same side

ischaemia   lack of blood supply to an area of tissue

Jacksonian epilepsy focal seizure involving the upper limb

Jacksonian march a seizure that starts focally in the hand, but spreads up the limb and often ends in secondary generalization

Kayser–Fleischer rings rings of brown pigment seen in the eyes of patients with Wilson's disease

Kernig's sign pain in the back associated with resistance to straightening a flexed leg due to meningeal irritation

Kveim test emulsified lymph node from a patient with sarcoid is injected intradermally into the test patient (you could not make this up). If positive a granuloma forms

La belle indifference apparent indifference to catastrophic illness

lacune small lake in Latin; now used for a small stroke, usually due to occlusion of an arteriole

lamenectomy decompressive operation on the spine where the roof of the spinal canal is removed

lateral geniculate nucleus a nucleus in close proximity to the thalamus through which visual input from the chiasma is relayed

lemnisci sensory tracts that decussate in the brain stem

leucocytosis an increased number of white cells

Lhermitte's sign actually a symptom; subjective feeling of paraesthesiae in the limbs or electricity down the spine brought on by flexing the neck; seen in cervical cord pathology, especially MS

limbic system structures thought to be important in emotion including the hippocampus, cingulate gyrus and hypothalamus

Machado–Joseph disease autosomal dominant ataxia

macula area of the retina with the highest concentration of cones, responsible for colour and acuity

magnetic resonance imaging (MRI) if protons are aligned with respect to their magnetic properties in a strong magnetic field, when that field is relaxed the signal produced by the protons as they revert to their natural state can be used to provide an image of the state of those protons

mannitol osmotic diuretic

masseter muscle used to close the jaw

meatus opening or passage

medial longitudinal fasciculus (MLF) white matter tract in the brain stem linking the VIth and IIIrd cranial nerve nuclei

median nerve nerve that supplies the thena side of the palm and some thena muscles

medulloblastoma aggressive glioma of the cerebellum, usually in children

Ménière's disease disorder of the inner ear characterized by deafness, vertigo and tinnitus

meningioma commonest benign brain tumour derived from the meninges

mesencephalon mid brain; the bit between the pons and the forebrain

metastasis lump of cancer spread from a distant site

micturition passing urine

milieux intérieur internal environment, temperature, oxygenation, nutrients, etc.

miosis pupil constriction

monocytes type of white cell

mononeuritis one nerve damaged

monoplegia paralysis of a single limb

monozygotic twins genetically identical twins

myalgic encephalomyelitis (ME) synonym for chronic fatigue

myasthenia gravis autoimmune condition of the neuromuscular junction characterized by fatiguability

mycoplasma pneumoniae a cause of atypical pneumonia

mycotic aneurysm dilation of vessel wall due to infection

myelin insulation round nerve cells that facilitates saltatory conduction

myelitis inflammation of the cord

myelogram X-ray of the spinal canal requiring contrast agent to be injected intrathecally (by lumbar puncture)

myelopathy cord disorder

myoclonus brief jerk of muscles resulting in movement of a body part

myodil oil-based contrast agent once used for myelograms

myopathies   muscle disease often endocrinological in origin, e.g. Cushing's myopathy

myositis   inflammatory disease of muscle. The two commonest are dermatomyositis and polymyositis

myotomes   embryologically derived segments of muscles

myotonia   tonic muscle spasm with slowness in relaxation

neocortex   the brain's most recent evolutionary addition and largest component of the cerebral hemispheres

neuralgia   painful nerve as in trigeminal neuralgia

neuroanatomy   anatomy that relates to the nervous system

neuroaxis   the central nervous system, brain and spinal cord

neuroectodermal   referring to the dermal origin of many of the supporting cells in the CNS

neuroepithelial   line of cells that are derived from embryological ectoderm

neurofibroma   benign tumour of Schwann cells

neurofibromatosis   genetic disorder with growth of Schwannomas on peripheral nerves also known as von Recklinghausen's disease

neuroimaging   methods of obtaining pictures of the neuroaxis, usually CT or MRI

neuroleptic   major tranquillizer, e.g. chlorpromazine

neuromythology   those theoretical constructs which are known to be false, but are necessary to make sense of the neurological world

neurone   nerve cell; neuron

neuropathy   damage to nerves

neuropraxis   damage to a nerve without severing the axons – usually compressive

neuroscience   the scientific study of the brain, the rest of the nervous system and muscle

neurosis   minor psychiatric illness, such as anxiety or conversion disorder, as opposed to major psychiatric illness, e.g. psychosis

neurotrivia   the concern of the small-minded and membership examiners

nodes of Ranvier   areas free from myelin

sheath on an axon where depolarization occurs

nucleus pulposus   squishy bit in the centre of an intervertebral disc

nystagmus   jerky, repetitive movements of the eyes

obtundation   reduced level of consciousness

oculocephalic reflex   deviation of the eyes to either movement of the head or cold stimuli placed in the external auditory canal

oculogyric crisis   involuntary upward deviation of the eyes

oligoclonal bands   polyclonal bands of immunoglobulin synthesis which if confined to the CSF is supportive evidence of a diagnosis of MS, but can occur in other conditions

oligodendrocyte   cell in the CNS that produces myelin

oligodendroglioma   tumour of the oligodendrocytes

opisthotonic   extensor spasm of the spine

orthostatic hypotension   low blood pressure brought on by standing up

orthostatic pneumonia   pneumonia due to immobility. Sections of lung can collapse and secretions accumulate, becoming infected, unless the patient moves and fully expands their lungs

oscillopsia   the subjective perception of nystagmus

papilloedema   swelling of the optic discs usually due to raised intracranial pressure

papule   spot on the skin, between 0.1–1 cm in diameter

paraesthesia   abnormal cutaneous feeling, e.g. pins and needles

paramedian pontine reticular formation (PPRF)   lateral gaze centre in the pons

paraparesis   both legs weak

paraphasic error   error in speech where a word is misspoken in a linguistic sense (either semantic or phonetic)

paraplegia   both legs weak/paralysed

parasagittal   parallel to the midline

paraspinal   by the side of the spinal column

parenchyma   substance of an organ (brain)

pathognomonic   characteristic of only one diagnosis

penetrance in genetics refers to the degree a gene is expressed

persistent vegetative state the lights are on, but no one's home – continuing state in which brain-stem functions are maintained, but higher cortical activities are lost

petechial 1 mm bluish scattered lesions on the skin

Phalen's sign paraesthesiae in the hands due to carpal tunnel syndrome on extreme extension of the wrists

phenomenologist person (usually a neurologist) who studies the phenomena (outward expression) of disease and behaviour

Phineas Gage man who accidentally damaged his frontal lobes and had a change of personality

photophobia intolerance of light

phylogenetically evolutionary; traces of our evolutionary development are present throughout our body systems. When the newer systems fail the more primitive systems may become apparent

plantar reflex response of the toes to a noxious stimulus to the sole of the foot (normally the great toe flexes)

pleocytosis increase in the number of white cells in the CSF

plexopathy dysfunction in a nerve plexus

plexus (brachial and lumbosacral) spaghetti junction of peripheral nerves, between the nerve roots and the nerves that lead into the limbs

polymerase chain reaction (PCR) method of amplifying the amount of genetic material

polymorphs polymorpholeucocytes, a class of white cells associated with bacterial infections

polymyositis inflammatory myositis

posterior at the back

posterior column white matter tract up the back of the spinal cord traditionally thought to carry vibration and proprioceptive information

postganglionic the nerves between the ganglion and the end organ

postsynaptic after the synapse

praxis the practical knowledge of how to do something

presyncope the feeling of cerebral hypoperfusion prior to loss of consciousness

preganglionic the nerves between the CNS and a ganglion

pressor producing a rise in blood pressure

presynaptic before the synapse

prion infectious agent made of protein which is associated with CJD

prolactinoma tumour of the pituitary that secretes prolactin

pronate rotate so the back is in an inferior position – forearm

proprioception perception of the position and movement of limbs

prosody the melodic component of speech

proximal near; c.f. proximal myopathy – muscles of shoulder and pelvic girdles affected more than hands and feet

pseudohypertrophy enlargement of muscle bulk, but without increased strength, initially seen in Duchenne muscular dystrophy

ptosis drooping of the eye lid

purpuric small 2–5 mm lesions on the skin

putamen a nucleus in the basal ganglia

quadriparesis all four limbs weak

quadriplegia all four limbs weak/paralysed

radial nerve nerve that supplies extensors in the forearm and a small area of skin at the base of the thumb on the dorsal side of the hand

radicular pertaining to nerve roots

radiculopathy disorder of nerve root(s), i.e. that part of the nerve from the spinal cord to the plexus

ramus a branch; in the nervous system the ventral and dorsal rami form the nerve roots

Renshaw interneurones small neurones in the spinal cord

repolarize regain the resting potential

resectable able to be taken out surgically

reticular formation loose collection of neurones in the brain stem responsible for arousal amongst other things

risus sardonicus spasm-induced smile

Rolandic fissure the central sulcus dividing the frontal from the parietal lobes

Romberg test the patient stands with the feet together and eyes closed. Inability to do this suggests proprioceptive failure. I was told in the USA that the British Army devised this test to identify those soldiers with tabes

rostral   towards the head (upwards)

saccadic eye movements   rapid eye movements from one target to another

sagittal plane   bisecting the body into right and left halves

saltatory transmission   method of transmission along myelinated nerves whereby the depolarization jumps from node of Ranvier to node of Ranvier

Schwann cell   cell in the CNS that makes the myelin sheath

scotoma   localized area of visual loss

sella turcica   bony hole in which the pituitary lies

sensory-neural hearing loss   deafness due to damage to the cochlea or the VIIIth cranial nerve, as opposed to conductive hearing loss

sepsis   infection

Snellen chart   test of visual acuity

spasticity   increased tone as seen in upper motor neurone lesions

spinocerebellar ataxia type 1   autosomal dominant ataxia

spinothalamic tract   white matter pathway from the spine to the thalamus carrying pain and temperature information

spondylolisthesis   displacement of one vertebrae upon another in an anterior/posterior plane

spondylosis   vertebral degeneration

spongiform encephalopathy   rare encephalopathy with spongy change in the brain (e.g. CJD)

stellate ganglion   ganglion at the top of the sympathetic chain

stenosis   narrowing

stereotactic   the use of three-dimensional coordinates to locate a lesion as in stereotactic surgery

sterognosis   the ability to recognize objects by exploring them by sense of touch

stylomastoid foramen   hole in the skull out of which emerges the facial (VII) nerve

subacute combined degeneration of the cord (SACD)   myelopathy caused by B_{12} deficiency

subarachnoid   under the arachnoid, between the arachnoid and the pia mater

subluxation   slipping on top of another, as in vertebrae

suboptimal   less than ideal

sulcus   the groove between gyri

superior   above

supinate   rotate so the back is in a superior position – forearm

synapse   junction between nerve and muscle or nerve and nerve

syncope   fainting

syringobulbia   syrinx extending into the brain stem

syringomyelia   progressive cavitation of the centre of the spinal cord

syrinx   cavitation of the spinal cord or brain stem

systemic lupus erythematosus (SLE)   autoimmune connective tissue disease, which frequently affects the nervous system

tachycardia   fast heart rate

temporomandibular joint   joint between the jaw and the skull

tentorium   from the Latin tent. A layer of dura that separates the posterior fossa (i.e. cerebellum and brain stem) from the middle fossa. There is a hole in it through which the brain stem meets the rest of the brain

teratogenic   has the propensity to produce abnormal babies

tetanic stimulation   many action potentials arriving one after another

tetany   muscle spasm usually due to a low ionized calcium

thalamus   major sensory and other systems relay station in the centre of the brain. Probably the seat of the soul

thenar eminence   fleshy part of the palm at the base of the thumb

thermoregulation   control of temperature

thoracotomy   opening the chest

thrombosis   a blood clot forming in a blood vessel

thymoma   usually benign tumour of the thymus

tics   brief twitches partially under voluntary control

Tinel's sign   paraesthesia in a median nerve

distribution on percussion over the carpal tunnel

tinnitus sound in the ear which is not real and is usually continuous

tomography an image obtained by combining views from many sectors

torticollis twisting of the neck into an abnormal posture

toxoplasma protozoal parasite which causes cerebral abscesses, particularly in HIV infection

tracheostomy opening the trachea to the skin

transect cut across

transverse across

tremor rhythmical repetitive movements

trigeminal nerve the Vth cranial nerve, which supplies sensation from the face, made up of three divisions; hence its name

trismus tonic spasms of the jaw

ulnar nerve nerve that supplies the ulnar border of the palm and most of the intrinsic hand muscles

uncus end of gyrus parahippocampus in the medial temporal lobe

uniocular one eye

VDRL Venereal Disease Research Laboratory – screening test for syphilis

Valsalva coughing, straining, vomiting; manoeuvre that raises intra-thoracic pressure

vasculitis inflammation of blood vessels

vasoconstriction narrowing of blood vessels

vasodilation widening of blood vessels

vasogenic from blood vessels

vasovagal syncope episode of loss of consciousness due to parasympathetic overactivity

vegan purist vegetarian who avoids all animal products

ventral front

vermis Latin for a worm, an apt description for the middle bit of the cerebellum

vertebra one of the 33 bones forming the spinal column

vertigo the subjective sensation of either the world or yourself moving usually in an axial rotatory fashion

vesicles small intracellular bags in the neurological context usually containing neurotransmitter

vestibular system balance system which involves the semicircular canals, vestibular nerves and brain-stem nuclei

viraemia viruses in the blood

visuospatial neglect inattention, usually towards one side

vitiligo autoimmune disease causing areas of loss of pigmentation

Vogot–Koyanagi–Harada syndrome recurrent meningitis associated with iridocyclitis and depigmentation of hair and skin

WR Wassermann reaction – a complement fixation text for syphilis

Wegener's granulomatosis rare necrotizing vasculitis

Wernicke's area area of parietal cortex at the top of the Sylvian fissure, usually on the left, involved in language

Wolf–Parkinson–White syndrome tachyarrhythmia due to an accessory pathway which bypasses the normal atrioventricle node

xanthochromia yellow discoloration in CSF due to breakdown products of blood

X-linked spinal and bulbar muscular atrophy (Kennedy's syndrome) progressive neuromuscular disorder in males with partial androgen insensitivity

ZN stain Ziehl–Neelsen stain, classical stain for TB, now superseded

Zimmer frame lightweight aluminium walking frame

Index

Make your training easier with...

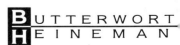

Pocket Companion to
Neurology in Clinical Practice, Second Edition

Iter G Bradley, D.M., F.R.C.P., Professor and Chairman,
Department of Neurology, University of Miami School of Medicine,
mi; Chief, Department of Neurology, Jackson Memorial
Hospital, USA

Robert B Daroff M.D. Chief of Staff and Senior Vice President
Medical Affairs, University Hospitals of Cleveland, USA

Gerald M Fenichel M.D. Professor of Neurology and Pediatrics
Chairman, Department of Neurology, Vanderbilt University
Medical Center, Nashville, USA

C David Marsden D.Sc., F.R.C.P., F.R.S. Dean and Professor of
Neurology, Institute of Neurology, The National Hospital for
Neurology and Neurosurgery, London, UK

- **Packed full of the clinical essentials contained in**
  Neurology in Clinical Practice, Second Edition
- **Portable, pocket-sized, and practical**
- **Quick and easy to consult**
- **User friendly access: abridged text and 160 tables
  plus appendices**

0 7506 9787 3   712pp   100 x 180 mm   9 illustrations
160 tables   Paperback   October 1996   £35.00

---

rder form

Qty   Title   ISBN   Price

Please add postage at £3.00 for UK, £6.00 for Europe, £10.00 for Rest
of World

Overseas customers: please pay by credit card or by cheque drawn in
sterling on a UK bank.

1. CHEQUE
Remittance enclosed £ _____
Cheques should be made payable to Heinemann Publishers Oxford

2. CREDIT CARD
Please debit my credit card as follows:

☐ Access/Mastercard   ☐ Switch   Issue No. _____

☐ Amex   ☐ Diners Start Date _____

☐ Barclaycard/Visa

Credit Card No:

Expiry Date:

NAME (PLEASE PRINT):

ORGANIZATION:

STREET: TOWN:

COUNTY: POSTCODE:

COUNTRY: DATE:

SIGNATURE:

DATE